AN IRISHMAN'S DIET

First published in 2008 by
Liberties Press
Guinness Enterprise Centre | Taylor's Lane | Dublin 8
Tel: +353 (1) 415 1224
www.LibertiesPress.com | info@libertiespress.com

Liberties Press is a member of Clé, the Irish Book Publishers' Association.

Trade enquiries to CMD Distribution
55A Spruce Avenue | Stillorgan Industrial Park | Blackrock | County Dublin
Tel: +353 (1) 294 2560
Fax: +353 (1) 294 2564

ISBN: 978–1–905483–16–7

2 4 6 8 10 9 7 5 3 1

A CIP record for this title is available from the British Library

Cover design by Dermot Hall
Internal design by Liberties Press
Set in Palatino

Printed in Ireland by
Colour Books | Baldoyle Industrial Estate | Dublin 13

An Irishman's Diet
A Marathon, Not a Sprint

Paul O'Doherty

LIBERTIES

To the Conscience and love of my life, Lorna

CONTENTS

INTRODUCTION

This is really hard for me to say, but here goes. My name is Paul O'Doherty and I'm an unhealthy-looking forty-something with a bulging compacted stomach and a chin that could have doubled as a lifeboat on the *Titanic*. Hovering at 18 stone, I've a 42-inch rope-a-dope waist that feels at times as if Angelo Dundee has loosened the epithelial tissues on my skin, and my stomach, liver and other internal organs are bouncing off each other like Ali and Foreman. The worst culprit is my liver, digging into my side, poking all the right nerves, teasing me about my size – a hernia-fest stuck in the airbags between my epidermis and internal organs. Not that my pains loiter exclusively around the cliff-face under my chest. Definitely not: my problems run much deeper. For every rumble in the jungle of my belly, there are the constant creaks, ailments and lingering pains in my back, legs, arms, armpits, chest, knees, arse, ankles and legs. I've even got a pain in my face: some sort of nerve ending that tiptoes under the right-hand side of my nose like a spot politician canvassing for acne outside a pus church. And if that wasn't enough, the World Health Organisation is sending up a flag that men with 40-inch waists should be hiding under the bed in fear of diabetes and writing to Santa Claus for a waistband that dances below 37 inches. Reluctantly, and a little scared, I think it might be just the time for me to embrace a diet.

Before I start, a few confessions. Firstly, two deep-rooted worms live in separate compartments of my body, one in my brain and the other in my stomach, and have a telepathic capacity to communicate the notion that fast food should be served in gigantic portions, morning, noon and night. And that chocolate, biscuits and cake are the only other super-foods worth eating. It's also a communiqué that I am loath to interrupt.

Secondly, I'm no one's fool and am completely aware that my Achilles heel – indeed the bane of my entire life – is my relationship with food and the amount of saturated and hydrated fat, added salt and spare sugar which lends itself to my normal diet.

Thirdly, keeping with the bumbling Achilles analogy, despite my love of chips, wedges, hamburgers and anything else that comes fast and fried, I know I'm doomed to an early death – although, I must confess, I'm not sure about the arrow to the heel, and the implication that Paris will kill me if I don't change. Anyway, to quote the vernacular, it's time for regime change. Time to dump the stodgy Hermann Göring-style frame that I've embraced since my youth. More Heinrich Himmler or Reinhard Heydrich than Pol Pot or Benito Mussolini – though without the politics and the uniforms, you understand.

Just to go back a stage, the Hermann Göring analogy is particularly apt in that Göring's diet in Nuremberg, according to Colonel Burton C. Andrus, the prison commandant at that infamous lodging house, 'made a man of him'. Andrus maintains that, when Göring arrived at the prison, 'He was a simpering slob with two suitcases full of paracodeine pills. I thought he was a drugs salesman.' Not that this pseudo army-cum-prison diet should be mistaken for the historically named Diet of Nuremberg, also called the Imperial Diet, which, according to the Golden Bull of 1356, every Holy Roman Emperor had to hold after his election. Since I'm not religious, this isn't really a runner (probably an inappropriate turn of phrase) for me, even if they do decide to bring back the title 'HRE'. And before you imagine going to all that trouble to be king, only to have some snivelling under-servant serve you a bowl of lettuce and a stick of carrot in Germany, 'diet' in this sense means 'deliberative assembly'. Those of you who know their Japanese politics will be aware that the Kokkai – the Japanese parliament – is known as the 'Diet' in English. Amazing how the word 'diet' drifts in and out of language.

All that aside, I'm not sure that the Nuremberg Diet, as Göring knew it, is a candidate either. The thought of getting involved in a beer-hall putsch, building Kernan-hall in honour of my wife (my wife's surname is Kernan; Göring named his home Karinhall, after his first wife), and then going into exile before returning, dressed as an albino baby elephant with a field marshal's baton the size of Louth, and burning down the council offices and contributing to the next great mass murder just isn't my style. Anyway, the way world politics has gone lately, it's probably easier to lose weight than to be convicted of crimes against humanity. And aside from all that, the thought does cross my mind from time to time that if I never lost the weight, I could go to acting school and become a method actor, specialising in roles for Latino dictators. Let's face it, it's not the most competitive of careers. Other than Bob Hoskins and Danny de Vito, how many fat-arsed, dumpy-faced actors are there?

Fourthly, I'm what I would call a moderate drinker who probably drinks too much. And lastly, I'm the most miserable individual this considerable side of the hamburger mountain. If I have a medical condition, it could probably be explained as Big Eyes, Big Mac, Big Arse syndrome. The thing is: I want to do something about it.

Now, this late-winter early-spring confession and mantra isn't unusual for me. I get these thoughts every winter, when any Michelin man worth his salt has to face up to the advent of the summer holidays – and natural exposure. It is, of course, a well-known fact that during winter fat people, to paraphrase Charles Lamb in *New Year's Day* – seeing as this is a new beginning of sorts – enjoy an immortality: we can hide behind the wind and rain in our long macs, stupid hats and French-tied scarves. That is, if we bother to go out at all. But no sooner has the odd bit of St Patrick's Day heat hit the ground than hiding places are at a premium. Suddenly, clothes loiter around the body like skin on a stuffed, pulled turkey, and dressing yourself is about as comfortable as decorating a bundle of loot with brown envelopes in a planning office.

Mornings are the worst, when what-am-I-going-to-wear-today?' type questions gallop like marauding insurgents around the bedroom, encircling and mocking the podgy, mountainous and blubbery cheeks that sit beanbag and Buddha-like astride my one-storeyed and squashed Pisa-tower excuse for a neck. Frequently, I sit on my side of the bed, short legs swinging like a ventriloquist's dummy, looking stupidly into the dark, cavernous wardrobe while the music from *Countdown* shell-shocks around the room, and ask, contestant-like: 'Go on, Carol, give us a shirt, a trouser and a vest.'

I ask in vain. This is a pity, because I love clothes. Or *used* to love clothes. That was, before I put on so much weight that I couldn't be bothered. I have now replaced fashion with necessity. In fact, shopping for clothes is a bit of a sensitive issue for me. Best to do it fast and at night, under maximum cover. My typical shopping day is planned with a nod to the annals of the military academy at West Point, Napoleon's mastery at Austerlitz, and Rommel's infantry blitzkriegs. Seal-like, I try to make my way into a shop, check the size on a pair of trousers, pay for them, and leave, all in one continuous motion, before anyone can get a glimpse of the Seven Bellies trying on the new parachute from Ralph Lauren.

Shopping isn't my only problem. Currently, I live and breathe in two pairs of trousers and two long-armed shirts, all blue and all moderately modern. I wear one set for good wear, special nights out, funerals and weddings, while the other, closer to me than my soul, is my de facto everyday uniform. Conscious that fat people smell more than thin people, I wash my live-in pair every day. This over-washing has caused a slight tear in the underbelly of my trousers and has made it impossible for me to wear even remotely bright jocks. This is all pretty miserable, because my wardrobe, and spare wardrobe, are full of trousers and shirts, waiting for the great day when I lose weight. At last count, I had a total of twenty-three pairs of trousers and twenty-four shirts. Good threads, you understand, not your usual rubbish that some fat people wear. Most of my gear is timeless. The best of quality bought in the sales, with the usual 'I'll look the business wearing that shirt when I lose four stone'.

Depressed, saddened and hurt, I'm as moody as any overweight footballing boy wonder. But not for long, for as soon as I finish this Southern-fried chicken and these crispy overcooked chips, I'm starting a diet.

JANUARY

THE DIET BEGINS: DIET CLASSES

Early January, and the low winter sun is raising its hat ever so slightly. The days – if you want to be mathematical – are getting longer. The early buds are promising daffodils and tulips, and the body, mind and soul are focused on being two stone lighter by March, four stone lighter by the summer, and a new man by next Christmas. And, as they say, I'm up for it. Up for it in the sense that I've convinced the head, mind, subconscious, unconscious and bejaysus that it's about time we did something about this. About time we went back to being the person we were, before the troubles. About time we sold out to the other side. Walked across the Rubicon to the healthy brigade – the boring people who eat sensibly and who, we're told, are happier, more popular and better-looking, get all the jobs they want, and can walk proudly into a chipper and order whatever they want without the person behind the counter looking back at them and repeating their order, sucking the enjoyment from their feast like Stasi food police. 'Three burgers, did you say? Separate or all together?' Why do they ask? They know they're all for me. Of course, they're having a dig. Next time you're in a chipper, listen out for whether the server asks a thin person 'Separate or all together?' No, they bloody well don't. They just can't help discriminating against the fat bloke.

Anyway, a newspaper report suggests that 'Two-thirds of men in Ireland are overweight, and 44 per cent are in denial' – according to the Irish Cancer Society. Luckily, at least for the moment,

11

I'm not one of them – in denial, I mean. Although the thought occurs to me that if I'm in denial, I probably don't know it. So, am I in denial? It's a bit like suggesting through the psychoanalysis loop that I'm conscious of my unconscious, which presumably I'm not. It also makes you wonder how they carried out the research. Did they ask the people whether they were in denial or not? And were the people who responded lying when they said they weren't in denial, or did they just not know that they were in denial in the first place? Like how the fuck do you measure denial?

Anyway, in denial or not, I'm on a diet, all 18 stone of me. I'm prepared to do what needs to be done to shed the belly, the extra chins and the tightness around the crotch. Initially, I'm aware that it's all bluster and motivational ring-tones, but honestly, I really believe that this time it's going to work.

So, three, two, one, starting at midnight on the first of January, I'm on the wagon. I wake hungry, although breakfast comes and goes without a problem. But then again, the old get-up-fill-up in the morning has never been a problem. I'm not a lover of porridge, and years ago I devised a breakfast cereal for oat lovers who hate that horrible grunge, which is either too lumpy or too watery: three big spoonfuls of oats, half an orange, half a kiwi, half a pear, half an apple, and something else in season – mango is a favourite – and then two or three spoonfuls of yoghurt, and half a passion fruit on top to spice things up, so to speak. You might wonder why I never use milk or hot water on my cereal. The truth is that milk and myself don't get on, for some stupid reason that probably goes back to my childhood. The thought of putting anything watery on my cereal is enough to have me retching.

No, my food-addiction problems tend to kick in mid-morning, when the breakfast, although satisfying (a new word in my vocabulary) and quite filling, starts to ask one or two questions of the senses, usually on the topic of: when's dinner? On a normal morning, it's going to be one of two scenarios: do you give in to temptation and park the diet, or do you grind your teeth and persevere? It's like having Jeremy Paxman in your head orchestrating an argument with his doppelgänger. Yes, you know it's good for you. Yes, you know it should do you through to lunchtime. And yes, if you're going to lose weight, you have to stop snacking. But goddamn it, I need something to eat. So what do I do? *Answer the question.* I don't know. *Come off it, answer the question.* I said I don't know. *Come off it, who are you kidding? Answer the bloody question. You're the one on the big fancy diet. What are you going to do?* You want to tell Paxo he's not so quick with his fancy quiff, but the quiff's on the other scalp this time.

The psychology of this conundrum comes down to the weighing scales of convenience. Initially, you go for a walk, anywhere, to keep your mind off the inevitable. Then your motivation hits a flat spot. You scour the office, the fridge, under the bed, the garden, or the children's sweet-box for a panacea that doesn't look like it's high in fat or has carbohydrates emblazoned on the wrapper. Ideally, you're looking for something with a bit of oomph, that's been through some rigorous SAS-style boot camp, and that tastes like heaven and will make you look and feel slimmer. By the time you realise that such items don't exist, your mind is alive with a UN resolution permitting interventionist action with complete plenipotentiary powers that will allow the self one grilled sausage followed by one chocolate biscuit provided that the self goes for a three-mile jog afterwards. *Deal!* you shout. *I'm on for that. Come on, vote! I said I'd do it.* The vote is positive. And before all the votes have been counted, a grill has been commandeered and is ablaze with four sausages, and you've eaten three chocolate biscuits while you were waiting. Bang. The diet's in free-fall, but you don't care. Afterwards, you're going to go for the mother of all runs. You're going to sweat like you've never sweated before, and your body, wife, dog, cat and the whole United Nations is going to be proud of you. You're going to be so good, no one will recognise the muscular, toned superman who's just left his outer shell.

Two hours later, you've had lunch: a big salad with wicked dressing, chicken wings, extra chips and half a bottle of house wine. You make your way back to work, full, annoyed with yourself, and angry that you couldn't say no. You refuse to make eye

13

contact with mirrors or reflections in shop windows. You hope you meet no one you know. You're ashamed that you've eaten like a pig and all you have to show for it is a heavy countenance and an even heavier stomach. A voice in your head mentions the UN resolution. Your broken promises, your diet, your desire to lose weight, and the early-evening run? You try to ignore them. Doesn't everybody? You rationalise your behaviour: I've done it, I'm ashamed of it, and I won't do it again. Halfway through the day, the diet is over.

Later that evening, you've plans to go out. The clothes issue shows up with a big, self-important question mark, its arms folded like it's seconds away from crying and ramming every argument for proper living down your throat. *What do I wear?* While shaving, your face looks back out from the mirror, podgy with another day's dinner or pig-out. You blame the chips, the chicken wings and the salad. A wash later, you stand by the mirror, and you've nothing that fits you. The one pair of trousers you wear on social occasions is tight, your belly isn't prepared to sit meekly back in the pew behind your belt, and your head is arguing the whole issue of diet by faith alone and the chances of nailing ninety-five theses to the fridge to remind you of your present misery every time you think of food. It's as if Martin Luther is hiding behind your leather belly-catcher, shouting the kernel of any decent schism: the art of indulgences – or over-indulgences. You wonder if Eisleben's finest had a problem with fat people. Maybe, maybe not. But then again, there was the Diet of Worms, where Emperor Charles V outlawed Luther as a heretic and made it a real no-no for anyone in Germany to offer him food or shelter. An unusual punishment, to say the least. Cause a schism in the Church, and they cut off your Nürnberger bratwurst and sauerkraut rations. Would it work today? Starvation instead of penalty points? Worth a try, I suppose.

Anyway, none of this helps your current predicament. You run your mind over Saddam Hussein's former hole. Is it available, or did the GIs dig it up and bury it where it could never be found? You have a fight with your wife. Yes, of course you want to go out, but, you plead, you've nothing to wear. The anger kicks in again and you promise: never, never again.

Dinner with friends is uncomfortable and, of course, while the sensibles from over the road are dodging the fat, salt and sugar with polite regret, you're the one who just can't be bothered. You're on a downward slide, so who cares? Might as well enjoy it. Walking home, to work off some of the excess, you begin the ritual again. Diet to start tomorrow at 8 AM. But it doesn't; it's Tuesday, you've another dinner to attend, and the thought of cheese meringues and roast potatoes is looming large in your mind. By Wednesday, it's the middle of the week, and too close to the weekend to begin anything. By the weekend, you've had more chips, a couple of takeaways, and lots of different bars of chocolate. On Sunday evening, you return your diet campaign to the cycle and plan for another attempt.

Reading over what you've written, you realise the *You* has taken over. Where is the *I*? In the course of the diary, *I* has become *You*, and blame has been shifted away from the self. It's an easy mistake to make. You – sorry, *I* – get to grips with it. Next week, I'll seek help with my diet.

The second week of the diet – or the attempt at a diet – suggests that help is needed. Not able to do it myself. Need a bit of willpower. Someone to hold my hand through the diet maze. So I join a men-only, self-help, we're-going-to-help-you-shed-the-pounds club.

I arrive on time. The room has all the hallmarks of a Stalinist waiting room: bare walls, drafts, dilapidated lighting and garish posters. The woman running the show meets me with the welcome. This is after I've joined up, paid my dues, taken off my coat and stood on the scales. We've met before, a year earlier, when I joined for one week, only to realise, as you do, that making a commitment to dieting and diet classes can impact a little more on your lifestyle than you care to admit. It's Groundhog Day for fat people. I weigh in at 18 stone 2 pounds. It's the heaviest I've ever been. The happy smile and the 'Sure we're going to help you' look don't hide the third eye that's welcoming a failure: an unhappy food-abuser who just knows that this isn't going to work.

I'm probably the youngest bloke in the all-male room, an assembly of different heights, waists and egos. The guy behind me smells. I guess he could shed a pound and a half if he washed. The bloke in front of me also smells. Body odour with cabbage. A thirty-something sits down beside me. Needless to say, he smells too. That's it, I can't move. Surrounded by blokes who hide their money under their bars of soap, I want to leave, but I rationalise that if this is the price for losing weight, I'm committed. There's also the realisation, from other personal anecdotes well in the past, that fat people all generally smell and dress appallingly: it's as though designer clothes don't exist for us. Some of the men in the congregation look as if they've slept in their clothes and are on day release from Guantánamo Bay, their orange jumpsuits at the cleaners. As noted already, I've been there myself: stuck with a minimalist wardrobe that at least actually fits.

I hear the guy behind me wheezing. He's out of breath: the gentle stroll up the stairs has nearly killed him. As I catch my own breath, two business-looking dudes arrive in suits. They could be consultants: blue suits, blue shirts and blue voices. They look like they're at the wrong convention. Another well-dressed younger chap arrives. He has the look of a guy getting married whose wife-to-be has chosen a wedding suit for him that's slightly too tight and has insisted that he go to diet school. He's not even married and she's making his sandwiches, has cancelled his subscription to Sky Sports, is vetting his friends and is replacing his designer labels with checks and country-house snobbery. In ten years' time, he'll be looking for his identity on a counsellor's sofa, wondering where it all went wrong. It crosses my mind that there should be bouncers on the door turning people like him away.

The class begins. The slim, well-dressed woman – the weight-management guru – tells us there are five types of eater: the nibbler, the muncher, the fast-foodie, the bulk-loader and the sweet-tooth. While some of the men take notes, I immediately think I'm all five. She asks the class: which are you? No one answers – not yet, anyway. She offers a few hints, and the feedback – not the most ideal of words – gathers momentum. Out of the woodwork storm the serial diet-classers. The lads with life stories – if not weight – to burn, who have presumably passed on the shrinks. The nibblers, the fast-foodies and the sweet-tooths (or should that be 'sweet-teeth'?) all have something to say. A self-confessed nibbler brings up the *Mona Lisa*, three of his favourite restaurants, and how Iraq was once called Persia. He talks so much, I'm surprised he has time to eat. I want to lean over and tell him that he could lose three stone in a week if he joined a debating society, but the guy with the cabbage aftershave is too close.

It's well-meaning chatter, and mostly entertaining. Everybody in the room is here because they share a common goal – to lose weight. And, looking around the class, success stories make themselves known with simple, well-meaning modesty. There are definite benefits to attending the session.

Eventually, the guru tries to wrestle back control of the class. She holds out a cake and asks the class: 'How many slices could you get out of this?' A sweet-tooth suggests seventeen. The guru is impressed. She holds up another cake – it's the same size as the first – and repeats the question. The sweet-tooth suggests nineteen. Again the guru is impressed. She holds up a third cake, the same size as the other two, and repeats the question. The sweet-tooth suggests four. 'Four?' she asks. 'Yes,' he says, 'that's my favourite.' The class laughs. It's like Bingo for fat people.

At the end of the class, the two consultants get stars and rocks for losing a stone each. I wonder if they're embedded food-abusers or food-abuser guru-inspectors, marking the guru out of ten. They're probably the thinnest people in the room, and definitely in the wrong place. Food-abuser spies, perhaps, from a rival organisation. Anyway, we clap and say goodbye like schoolchildren leaving school – and a favourite teacher – at the end of term. The serial diet-classers gather around the guru for private tuition. I leave as fast as I can, rejuvenated now that I've had an education. For the moment, anyway, thoughts of food couldn't be further from my mind.

*

We're nearing the end of January, and it's been an eventful first week on the managed diet. I'm now officially a fat bloke with a plan and a calorie-planner, and I've implemented one or two changes which I'm hoping will correct everything that's wrong with my life. I'm also beginning to think differently, redesigning my mindset, if not quite my body-shape. In other news, the slim, well-dressed weight-management guru has eloped with a Japanese wrestler and been replaced by Mr Enthusiastic himself, the most positive weight-manager in diet-land.

Having weighed in, the cheerful band of slimming brothers – Fat Troop, F-Troop, call us what you like – offer up inspiring tales of how they've lost five pounds, six pounds and seven pounds. I cringe when the septuagenarian (I kid you not) to my right informs us, having been coaxed on by Mr Enthusiastic, that the only morsel of fat that has passed his lips in five weeks is a slice of pudding on Christmas Day. I wonder sympathetically if the poor man believes that funeral directors will one day bury you by the pound and is trying to alleviate future funeral expenses. It seems rude to tell him I think he's out of his mind.

When it's my turn to glory in my miserable one-pound weight-loss, I'm embarrassed to make eye contact, especially when Mr Enthusiastic asks me to expand on 'my wonderful news'. Wonderful news? I feel like I'm the worst newsreader on the Humpty Dumpty channel. I try desperately to wriggle out of my awkward performance by arguing that, while I've physically lost only the bare minimum, psychologically I've lost stones in bad eating habits and inadequate exercise routines, and scorned the mind games of late-night chippers and other nibbles. F-Troop smile at me, knowingly, as I release the parachute of denial for the last time, their heads tilted like a mother offering a pitiful child a sigh of comfort. While I smile back affectionately through my clenched teeth, inside my competitive streak is in overdrive. I want to crush them all, to be the number-one weight-loss fat bloke ever. And to show this bunch of weight-losers that I'm just as good as them. Next week, I determine to show them a thing or two about slimming.

Indignant, I sit quietly for the rest of the class, marvelling at the genuine decency and achievement of seriously overweight

people glowing in their hard-earned reductions, having decon-
structed their humble roast dinners and morning fries, replacing
carbohydrate domination with vegetable balance. How people
change when smitten by the diet-class bug: it's no lie to say that
hardcore snake-oil salesmen have become poster boys for green
stir-fries. As the class ends, the weight-guru brings to our attention how few calories there are in Curly Wurlys. A few minutes
later, F-Troop pass me in a lather of sweat as I saunter up the street
to the local shop. By the time I get to the cash register to pay for
my paper, a bemused Chinese tells me 'The Curly Wurlys all
gone'. Panic-buying means that the chocolatey rope ladder is no
longer in stock. It's a Basil Fawlty moment. And if we'd ever gone
to war with China and won, I'm sure the Chinese would have
said: 'Whatever did you win?' It's also another personal failure
for me. Not only is F-Troop out-dieting me, they're also out-eating
me, out-pacing me and out-buying me.

Later, at home, the competitive spirit is pulsating around in
my brain like the recently relinquished demented war-drum that
once frogmarched me to the nearest chipper. I'm suddenly in the
results business: me, F-Troop and every other weight-watcher. I'm
the relegation-threatened bottom-of-the-table manager of the fat
division, and every fur-coated chairman living the dream is the
trigger-happy weighing scales. But now it's personal, and I'm
truly committed to dramatic change.

I decide to make soup. Soup, you say? Yes, soup. I search
around for a recipe, tripping through the exotica of Russian lemon
soup, peach and mango soup with coconut milk and yoghurt, and
German marrowfat-pea soup with sausage, amongst many others, before deciding on carrot soup, mainly because carrots are the
only vegetable left in the house in any quantity and I don't fancy
doing an evening shop. It's a simple recipe, one I've grown fat
avoiding and one that's probably available in some recipe book or
other. I throw an onion into our biggest pot, add a knob of butter
and a teaspoon of olive oil and allow the onion to sweat in the fat
for about ten minutes. I put the kettle on and pour hot water over
two ordinary vegetable stock cubes in a glass jug before adding a
shake or two of turmeric, paprika, cumin and cinnamon.

Allowing the ingredients to get to know each other, I chop up a sweet pepper, about ten carrots and two smallish potatoes. When the onion has sweated its brains out, I add the vegetable stock, the vegetables and the potatoes. I also add a cup of lentils to bulk out the mixture. After about an hour, the soup – vegetables floating in water – looks like Victorian prison rations and, aesthetically speaking, pretty damn disgusting. Tasting the unfinished product at this stage has often discouraged me from eating soup for months, so I dig out the hand-blender and machine-gun the lot, rotating the blender around the pot to break up all the orange pieces. Adding more pepper than salt, I sit down to an alternative evening meal that should keep me in nutrition for the next seven nights, determined to break new weight-loss records. Does home-made soup guarantee weight loss? Only, I suppose, if you eat it.

The seven days of soup-rationing works up to a point. I find it's OK when the soup is hot, preferably coming from the big pot. The problem is, I can't bear to be in the same room, town or country as soup when it's cold, even as it's being reheated. It smells, looks and slithers disgustingly. I can't even touch it when it's in the fridge. And obviously I'd cuddle rats before I'd stomach gazpacho. Somewhere in my unconscious there's a lever that's permanently set in the I-hate-cold-soup position, and no amount of psychology is going to change the situation. So I make enough soup to do myself and the missus for a week. The first day there's no problem because, well, it's warm from the cooker. And once I don't put the remainder in the fridge, the second day doesn't go so badly either – because I don't mind reheating it from the pot. By the third day, taking it out of the fridge is beyond me. The smell, liquidity and consistency are torture. No, brother, no can do. I'm like the novice hurdler who's just won a bumper by twenty lengths but can't adjust to jumping anything higher than a blade of grass.

That's not to say I give up, though. I decide to make smaller quantities of soup and eat it while it's still hot, occasionally playing around with the recipe, like grating the carrot or adding a leek. I also ask the wife, when she's around, to pull the psychological wool over my eyes and do all the transferring from the fridge to a hot plate when I'm not looking. I realise she's made warm soup from the cold preserve of the fridge when she calls me into the dining room for my dinner. That is, of course, on the days neither of us is at work. She also adds milk to the soup – to give it a creamy consistency. Did I mention that I don't like milk? Yes, the wife, without telling me or letting me see, adds milk to the heated soup to cool it. Yes, I know that sounds like madness, but that's women for you. Why don't they just not heat it up so much?

For the most part, the soup is all right, if a little time-consuming to prepare. It's not *not* called fast food for nothing. It also means that you have to be close to a kitchen for most of your existence. And don't try cooking soup near work colleagues if your kitchen happens to be on the same level as your workstation. How to lose friends and influence nobody immediately springs to mind. Likewise, if you can stomach the reheating gig, avoid reheating soup in the communal microwave, unless you work with people you don't like and you want to stink the bejaysus out of it for the next man or woman.

Of course, home-made soup shouldn't be mistaken for the branded alternatives that fill our supermarket shelves and come in round tins, shiny plastic packages or disposal cartons. Easy to buy, stack and cook with, they are tasty for the most part, and you can doctor them up with as much ammunition from the herb garden as you like. However, the better ones are as fattening as fast food and come laced with enough salt and extras to stockpile nuclear fat. They're also a hell of a lot dearer than the home-made varieties – not that I'm advocating that the cost should be a fat issue, of course.

February

Exercise and Health

By the start of February, the soup programme has reduced my gut by half an inch, although I still can't fit into my forty-inch downsize trousers and, as for movement on the scales, the baby finger doesn't look like it's moved in four weeks. The problem, I suppose, is getting distracted. In fact, four weeks into my diet, I think the single most important requirement for anyone contemplating weight loss is for them to be occupied. The French knew it, the Poles knew it, and now the Iraqis know it. Monotony is the enemy, ingratiating itself into your confidence, taking you for walks to the fridge or on fly-bys past the chipper and prompting the dreaded 'Jesus, I'm bored. Think I'll drive up to the Fast-food Reservation and liberate the Black Hills of Dakota's hamburger mountain'.

And, obviously, supermarket shopping is the meanest distraction of all. Yes, sir, outside the realm of the chipmakers' cartel, it's probably the worst reservation on earth. With six-odd weeks to St Patrick's Day and the first real hint of spring, a morning spent supermarket shopping on an empty stomach is lethal. Over the years there's one hard lesson I've learned: if you're going to pig out on fast food, chips or breaded Southern-fried chicken, don't do it at a supermarket. Overcooked, flavourless and often cold, such food is to be avoided. Better to buy the bloody ingredients and make some sort of a stab at a home-made dinner, served up, however gluttonously, to your own specifications. Fast food should never be left to others, particularly those working in Irish supermarkets. Remember: proper fast food is personal, local and a product of anti-globalisation.

Luckily for me, though, I've moved on. I'm thinking distraction. And so I've been occupied, relentlessly occupied, and by Jove I think it's worked. No more greasy cardboard-tasting hamburgers for you, I hear you say, and you're right. So, with a good breakfast under my chassis, it's on out for the weekly shop. I find myself loitering around the veggie department with soup on my mind. What do I find? Well, it's a little unpredictable. What you're looking for are those cute little veggies that don't look as if they've spent the early winter on sunbeds and the rest of the hibernatory period on extraordinary renditions – discoloured, soft, and on their deathbeds, the tears of their over-ripeness pouring unwanted juice on top of their fellow detainees. But you may as well be looking for a Taoiseach with a bank account. Where are all the buy-me flavoursome vegetables that seem to star only in recipe books? Is rubbery broccoli now a variety, and do cauliflowers naturally come with Ash Wednesday ashes?

You can't buy an onion without peeling away a confession box of sins, and as for potatoes, what's the problem with sourcing decent floury spuds? It's no wonder some people couldn't be bothered eating vegetables. And how much of what we buy regularly do we just add to our compost bins or browns bins at the end of the week? I suspect it's higher than the average householder admits. Is it 40 percent of our veggies? More. Was there a time recently when you bought a week's supply of vegetables in the one shop and didn't have to put them on a life-support system as soon as you got home. 'Doctor, doctor, I can't find a pulse, 1 over 100, I think we're losing the broccoli.' Yes, we've all been there.

Sick of rubbery broccoli, over-oranged carrots and bruised cauliflower, it's probably a good idea to buy from your local greengrocer or veggie baron, if you're lucky enough to live near one. However, where I live, there isn't one, certainly not within walking distance. So how do I eat fresh greens regularly? Well, you can't, can you? One of these days, next time I'm in my local supermarket, I'm going to peel every last vegetable at the till before I buy it, to make sure everything is in order. And apologies to anybody who's behind me in the queue, at the time, for the inconvenience. Not that I'm the only one thinking this way. I'm sure there are lots of people who would love to inspect their produce at the till before buying it and bringing it home, leaving skins, peels and yokes behind them, like any proper-minded green-shopper should be doing at the moment. How quick would the supermarkets then be to buy produce locally and in season, and reintroduce the meaning of freshness?

That's all very well, but it doesn't solve my problem at the moment. If I want to eat veggies every day, I have to buy them nearly every day. This involves commitment, and a regime designed for a professional green-shopper who is able to dedicate more than an hour a day to shopping. Even if I was in the Green Party, I wouldn't have time to do that – not least of all if I was in government and cycling to work every morning. And how many veggies would I be able to carry in my butcher's bicycle? And what's the alternative? Frozen veg? As Basil Fawlty says: 'Well, they were fresh when they were frozen.' So, standing in a supermarket with dead or dying vegetables, I bought enough frozen veg to sandbag a river. It must be noted that frozen veg or watery vegetables are usually tasteless and to be opened only in desperation. Nutritional value? I suppose you could live on them, barely.

Whatever the condition of the vegetables on supermarket shelves, generally speaking fruit is much better when it is preserved – although I'd hate to think that this was because of the quality of the preservatives instead of the quality of the fruit. Finding fresh pears, apples, kiwis and oranges well stocked and in good condition on the supermarkets' shelves is rarely a problem, even if mangoes in recent years are often over-ripe and too woody.

I'm now more than a month into the diet, and while I'm still a little less worried about my food intake, my health has taken a turn for the worse. Since the first week of February, I have been in nearly constant pain. What caused this mother of all ailments? Well, it's difficult to say. Difficult to say in the sense that my diet is a coalition of the willing, a roadmap to a better me, and involves everybody digging in and encouraging me to shed the pounds. And, as any agreeable coalitioner will tell you, you don't want to distance yourself from the minister for justice because you don't agree with everything he says, not if you're in a coalition that is a little abrasive and has a digestive system that is particularly suited to renditioning vegetables. That is, until there's a change of government and that particular official is replaced by someone else.

This hasn't really been the case with my disposition, although in a similar vein, it is difficult to ostracise any member of my little coalition of prunes, oats, carrots, tiny potatoes and all the various minuscule seeds I eat with my breakfast, even if one of them has a habit of being overly vigorous with its intended goodness. The trouble is that we've been infiltrated by a rough agent, possibly one of the seeds, who has holed up somewhere disagreeable between my lower stomach and the upper delta of my bum. How do I know? Well, my doctor said so. Constipated, suffering from backache, and feeling that *War and Peace* was being rewritten in my out-chute with a pencil the size of the Wellington Monument, the particularly invasive toilet evacuations, chapter-tome by chapter-tome, had me shuffling to the doctor like a scuba-diver trying to walk with a stretcher tied to his back. The doctor, having asked, incredulously, 'You've not eaten unground seeds, have yeh?', diagnosed a rectal tear, and prescribed a week's supply of suppositories and a gallon of laxative.

Five minutes later, down the road, the chemist's assistant handed over a rather large container of loosing agent, while the chemist discreetly passed me a box marked 'Insert rectally' and, lowering his voice, sympathetically enquired: 'Have you used these before?' While the suggestive and invasive nature of the King Kong-lettered 'Insert rectally' instruction gave the game away, the temptation to reply in the negative was balanced by the fact that, staring at the laxative like Pavlov's dog, I felt that a Dunkirk evacuation was imminent. The chemist's wasn't the appropriate place to be surrounded by Germans, metaphorically speaking, and there weren't enough tugboats to bring me back to

Blighty. Luckily, I made it home in time, although the chemist's assistant's time-delaying request for change of a €20 note was as deadly as any spiralling Stuka dive-bomber.

At home, the games really got going when, having swigged on the bum-loosener, I went about the delicate procedure of inserting the damn things 'rectally'. Now, I'm not sure whether this is the best place to discuss how a fat bloke with a wine barrel for a tummy, genuflecting, assuming the position, and holding on to the bath for dear life, tries to one-handedly insert an *Apollo 13*-shaped rocket up his lunar capsule with all the dexterity of a gymnast trying to stay within the confines of the horizontal bars. So I won't, save to say that, three hours later, and smelling of a compound of prednisolone and I won't say what, I felt what Buzz Aldrin must feel every day of his post-astronaut's life: all that bloody effort, and I'm still remembered as 'the second bloke to stand on the moon'.

Aside from all the medical mishaps, the good news is – and I'm not sure whether the soup or the embedded seeds deserves the Oscar – that I'm down a whopping half a stone, and now weigh 17 stone 7-ish. And I'm also down a trouser size, from a 42-inch waist to a 41. It's still parachute-class but it's progress. The only downside has been that they don't make trousers in 41-inch sizes, the trouser-land mandarins taking the view that fat people go up and down the scale in two-inch increments. So I'm stuck in my 42-inch navies, forcing the torque on the belt two notches down the line. Otherwise, it's been a slow five weeks and, while the bum situation has provided plenty of exhortation, it's probably a good time to take up something called exercise. I can't imagine what it's like but I'm looking forward to it.

It's at this time of year that I assess my annual underpants requirements and make the requisite purchases. Unfortunately, this year I dived in much too early and, before I'd had time to come to terms with any weight loss, foolishly bought trunk sizes. So I tried to do a bit of a Chelsea and get out of what you might call my 'sponsorship deal' and brought back my seventeen pairs of unused jockeys. However, the shop's 'We don't accept back used or unused jockeys' policy meant that, for the first week of my exercise campaign, I was kitted out in long-decommissioned jockeys that are possibly a notch tighter than required. Not that jockey size is the biggest bugbear for anyone with a weight problem taking up exercise. The fact is that fat blokes aren't supposed to exercise. It's a bit like cartooning the minister for health in a tracksuit, taking the honest stand against obesity. As anyone who has ever bought a tracksuit will tell you, fat people, despite the advice, from doctors, dentists and greyhounds not to wear a tracksuit, are perfectly within their rights to wear a tent, a garden shed or a Joseph-coat of umbrellas, but just dare them to don a pair of runners or dust down their old 1970s tracksuit with stripes down the side and go for a run . . . . Statistics have even shown that fat people are as popular in tracksuits as the West German police force were in their tracksuits at the 1972 Munich Olympics, although, for us, it's never just one day in September.

Nothing is going to get in my way when it comes to losing weight, though. And if the end justifies the means, I'm going to wear a tracksuit. I'm not afraid of being called a Machiavellian. So on the first day of my exercise campaign, I leave the house, my head set on a circuit of sorts. Within minutes, it's a brisk walk. I get a bit excited. Using a pair of grandparents pushing a perambulator as a pacemaker, I set off like a pregnant Mick the Miller on erythropoietin dressed head to toe in my white tracksuit, which, having run slightly in the wash, gives a slightly off-red glow – a little paler than a Teletubby, but not quite as dark as the Ready-Brek Kid.

People stare at me as I make my way up the road. I can see the amusement and derision in their eyes. Nods and titters of laughter to their colleagues and friends follow: 'Look, there's a fat bloke in a tracksuit.' I swing my arms and try to get the breathing right. The stares continue, and everyone seems to have a smile. As I build momentum, however, I notice the outside intrusions less and start to focus with the concentration of a world-beater.

This is easy, I say to myself, and break into an extended jog. It's the over-enthusiasm of a first day, and soon I'm bouncing up the road, dreaming of Olympic success. In my mind, I'm the oldest athletic ever to compete in three events at the Games. Minutes later, I'm overtaking five athletic-looking Africans. Three of them are possibly Kenyans, one of them's definitely a Moroccan, and is that really the great Ethiopian Haile Gebrselassie? I pass the bus-stop, the chemist's and the cemetery. It's world-record pace. The Africans are nowhere to be seen. Every post's a winning one. I'm bagging medals and running out of mantelpiece space. Soon, I've won gold in the 1,500 metres, the 5,000 metres and the marathon, and there's talk amongst the sportswriting corps that I'm to be named in the senior Irish squad for the forthcoming soccer internationals. That is, until disaster strikes.

It's the bloody underpants. Tight, a little restricted, and by this stage mauling the jewels, the fabric has tightened around the crevices of my groin. My flabby, overstretched flesh starts to rub against itself, and I can feel a rash doing altitude training in the Atlas Mountains nether-regions of my jockeys. The pain cuts a hole in my enthusiasm, and I stop. As the Africans catch up and pass me, I struggle with the mother of all elastics, pulling it this way and that, desperate to find an equilibrium that will allow me to finish the circuit, and even more desperate that everybody else walking their dog, cat, child or goldfish isn't mesmerised by the fatty walking sideways with the elastic from his jockeys forming a sliding perimeter round his thighs. It's not to be, however. I struggle home, my legs flung in front of me as if I've just gotten off the ghost of Red Rum without a saddle. I'm nearly crying with the pain and I curse the fact that, although I bought the petroleum jelly, put it on the table before I left the house, and even opened the damn lid, I forget to tool up – to cover my thighs, groin and wobbly bits in the jelly solution that I always plaster my legs with before I go for a walk.

Later, showered, and my creases, warts and bloodspots smothered in a blanket of antiseptic healing cream, I reflect on the fact that, though immobilised for the afternoon, I'm down another three pounds, to the stable weight of 17 stone 2. Seeds, underpants and pain – leftovers on the march towards slim-imity.

*

As any dieter will tell you, however, it's one day at a time, and lapses do occur. My first lapse comes in the middle of February, when I find myself struggling with the diet-management. It's seven-odd weeks since Christmas, and it's recession in weight-camp country, you might say. Everything was going fine until an end-of-the-week meal with some friends shoved temptation to the limit. And it wasn't as if I hadn't prepared as well as I could. I'd even built up a bit of an appetite by passing on the dinner-time soup and fat-loaded nibbles during an afternoon drive. Comfortable in my forty-inch trousers, I thought I looked the part as I accepted my first glass of Veuve Clicquot at the soirée. Bang. The diet was in free-fall.

I say free-fall, but that's probably an exaggeration. Like any of those pilots who tend not to fall asleep at the controls but who struggle perilously with the altimeter, I imagined myself taking the pressure off my diet and nosediving a couple of hundred feet, and parking it at the comfort zone, where weight is neither put on nor lost. For one night only, you understand. This wasn't a man out of control, but a mature slimmer with serious responsibilities. However, the voices of 'don't do it' started to throw a bit of a tantrum in my head and wouldn't accept that I was being measured, and that consenting adults – myself and the dietary advisors in my head – however aggrieved, could reach a compromise of sorts. So, sipping another glass of champagne, I set an example and initially passed on the flirting blinis – their whipped-cheese bods sunbathing in adorable sun-soaked oils on the biscuit-loungers. Then, in a moment of dementia, I could see in their pretty little eyelids the salutation of a thousand adorable cholesterol investments, fat-packed pensionable PRSAs and AVCs explained in the metaphor of food. Regrettably, I invested heavily and bit, as they say, of the apple.

The evening progressed and, another couple of yellow-bubbled glasses later, hunger came pounding at my door – mad, drink-induced and ravenous, if you know what I mean. Luckily, dinner arrived just then, and by the time seconds were being served, I was in my granny's. Later, it dawned on me how it's always easy to spot the fat bloke at a dinner party: he's the only one excessively encouraged to have more, and more, and more. 'A last roast potato', you hear. 'Sure you might as well have it – it'll only go to waste.' Weak and busted, you accept it, while everybody else around the table, in their slim-fitting chinos and designer T-shirts, gives that knowing nod and smile that tells you that, yes, you're an absolute savage – their little square fat friend in the tyre-vest.

You rationalise that you haven't done too badly. OK, so you've over-indulged and made a bit of a pig of yourself, but it's only one night, and tomorrow's another day, and it's all reparable, and sure why not have another couple of drinks as well to boot? It'll all be OK in the morning.

But it isn't. Tomorrow comes early and you're hungover and tired, and you haven't slept much. Never could sleep with too much food or too much drink. You know what's going to happen next. You pass on breakfast and start to fill up on cold fizzy drinks straight from the fridge – precisely the ones you haven't touched since the first week of the diet. It's cure time, and you're Dorothy running around with losers looking for the one-plan Wizard or any sub-prime loan to get you back to the good hamburgers of Kansas. And if Toto's not careful, you'll eat him and all.

However, a last modicum of dietary control lingers. You'll go for a walk. Where? Anywhere. To the toilet, the photocopier, or even round the block. Somewhere safe from the munchkins, or munchies, or whatever they're called. You go missing for seconds, minutes, half an hour, running anywhere away from temptation. To use a film analogy, it's the twenty-third century and you're Michael York in bloated Logan 5 apparel and, with a Jenny Agutter-type in tow, you're going to run, and as far away from the Sandmen of burgers, chicken nuggets, wedges, and all the other carbohydrates that the demon drink induces. It's sanctuary or bust. Lacking any conviction, you run down the nearest corridor but end up at the pig-out station – another day lost at the expense of the first. A day later, you pass on weight-class, F-troop and the probabilities of weight gain. Guilty to the tune of failure, and loaded with issues of absenteeism, you see in the mirror a coward's face rich with the blubber of excess, and a difficult week ahead to regain the hard-won ground.

Seven days later, you reflect on your restitution, that it's been a tough week in the weigh-loss bargain basement but you're back on an even stricter diet, and desperate once again to succeed. It's also confession time. Over the weeks, I've been fiddling around with the numbers, jumbling the figures, you could say, to make myself look good. It's Enron accountancy for fat people, diverting the food-intake amounts to imaginary offshore partnerships, defrauding the readership that I'm actually in better shape than I am. Nothing strong enough, you understand, to cause a Barings-like collapse in the weight world, but cheating nonetheless. Surprisingly, it wasn't the food. Or even the drink. Or even the exercise. No, I cheated on the weighing scales. And, if I'm really being honest, it was bloody easy.

Going back to my first class, I'd worn my heaviest socks and boots and an extra pair of vests, and filled my tent-size trousers with my two mobile phones, a plethora of household batteries, as much change as I could muster without noisily bringing attention to myself, and the odd bit of turf, and had lassoed two oblong-shaped paperweights around the elastic inside my underpants. Of course, my first weigh-in was exaggerated. This was handy when it came to accepting the plaudits from my F-troop colleagues as, over the weeks, I started to remove my stockpile of adjustments and appeared to be losing weight. Another trick I learned over the weeks was that, by positioning my feet on the fat-instructor's weighing scales in a certain way – putting the pressure on the edge of the scales – I got a more favourable reading.

But hey, that was in the past, and possibly last week's pig-out brought me to my senses, digging up enough of the old feelings of failure, uncomfortableness and personal hatred to jump-start another rehabilitation. So I've decommissioned all the batteries, the extra mobile phone, fertiliser, elastic and ton-weights, and embraced the policing authorities in fat-school. And I am prepared to distance myself from paramilitary hamburgers and wedges eaten on the run or otherwise, and to accept fully that the gun-man of overeating and lack of exercise has been for twenty-odd years the bane of my humpty-dumpty lifestyle. I'm also prepared to sign up to any policing scheme that will ensure my personal happiness for the next forty years. So this week I'm back on the wagon and motivated enough to undermine all those ego-posters that see the self as the poster boy for diabetics or that *Lost* lookalike Hugo 'Hurley' Reyes, with the $156 million weight problem. As a measure of my more honest and transparent regime, I've treated myself to a new weighing scales.

Of course, buying a weighing scales is never straightforward for a fat bloke. And, to the frustrated ironed-shirt Mr Angry with the lollipop tie who chastised me in a well-known department store with the inappropriate and overly loud-sounding 'Hey, you, if you break that, you'll have to pay for it', I can assure you that I'll never shop in your store again. What was I doing to elicit such a rebuke? Well, I was trying out weighing scales. Trying out weighing scales? Yeah, I didn't know how to try out a weighing scales either. That was until I read that British MP, agony aunt and *Celebrity Fit Club* participant Ann Widdecombe – who incidentally lost two stone on the programme – had tested five such inanimate objects for the *Observer*. I was particularly taken by her favourite – the Salter Mechanical Bathroom Scale – which the former Tory minister for prisons maintained had 'a pleasingly good-sized platform, and you could jump on it from a distance and it wouldn't slip'.

Now, I don't want you to think I'm the sort of bloke who wakes up in the morning and says to himself 'Jesus, I'm bored. I think I'll go down to the local department store and annoy the bathroom sales staff', but this opportunity sounded too good to be true. So at the weekend I went shopping for a weighing scales, specifically one that I could jump on from a distance. However, the good folk in a number of bathroom arcades in Dublin department stores had a problem with the idea of jumping on the weighing scales from a height, and under no condition was I allowed to run and jump. That was until I set up an experiment in one of the aisles which caught the attention of one particularly fussy department head, who told me in no uncertain language that yes, I could go and 'take a running jump' as he asked me to leave the store before he called security. The rules of caveat emptor – buyer beware – apparently don't apply to fat people.

I had to send in a plenipotentiary to buy the damn weighing scales, and she refused point-blank to test it for me before buying it. That's the problem with women – they just don't have any balls. But hey, that's more of a domestic altercation than a fat issue.

MARCH

THE ALLOTMENT

March is probably the scariest month for fat people – a sort of halfway house between the turkey-roll and ham-basted gluttony of Christmas and the naked appreciation of a sun-drenched Mediterranean beach. Scary in the sense that the temperature clock is ticking and by the end of the month you're likely to be wearing one less layer of clothing for longer periods, and that means one less layer of camouflage. So unless you have plans to go birdwatching in Bogotá or to engross yourself in the top-one-hundred must-see-before-you-die hide-and-go-seek destinations, you're going to be showing more (or less, if you've lost weight) of yourself, more often, in the coming weeks.

If you're a happy-meal new-year dieter, you should also be dreading the mid-term exams – a time around the Ides of March when you should have annihilated the Julius Caesar of all weight-problems and marched everybody into your office, court, senate – Mum, Dad, the daffodils, Octavius, Mark Antony and that know-all soothsayer – and proclaimed that you're at least halfway to reaching your target weight. Or maybe not? Maybe, like me, you still don't get the notion that over-eating is not good for you. *Et tu*, too much too?

But that's probably too much of a Roman generalisation. Personally, I've come to prefer an Eddie O'Sullivan-style of analysis. To paraphrase Ireland's greatest living mathematician, sorry, coach – statistically speaking, if you exclude the takeaways I've had every Wednesday and Thursday since I started the diet, and the first three weeks of January, or the slip I had on the Wednesday before Pancake Tuesday, I've had the caterers in from the local chippy or Indian emporium on fewer occasions than in the previous three months of other dietary campaigns. And if you turn a blind eye to my mid-morning-to-mid-afternoon performance in my last ten starts – again, statistically – I have eaten marginally less chocolate and sweets than a schoolroom of sweettooths.

But, not to blind you wholly with science, there have also been results. A whole stone of results, to be precise. Only a stone, you ask? Well, maybe next time when you're in the local supermarket during rush-hour, you might pick up a basket, fill it with fourteen one-pound butter-bricks and carry them around for a hour, and you'll get the opportunity to experience what the new me is beginning to enjoy every day. And watch the reactions of your fellow shoppers as you pile in the milk fat, and you might be some way to understanding what's it's like for a fat bloke to have fourteen of these missiles hanging from his pelvis every time he adds a stone to his burgeoning carcass.

Apart from the intermediate results, I've been good this week. 'Good' being fat-terminology for eating normally. I have been so good that I've set myself a goal. Well, actually two goals. Medically speaking, I have an appointment in the liver clinic in four weeks – fatty tissue apparently around the old boomerang-thingy – residue from hamburger hill and too many fat-clinging doggy bags. Again the clock is ticking, and my Middle Eastern doctors are expecting results. Promises, you understand, I made at the last appointment, when they laid it on the line for me. So I'm in serious training for blood tests in a few weeks.

My second goal is a mid-term break in France with the missus. With nothing to wear, and fearful that the temperatures are rising on the Gironde, I've promised myself and herself that I'm going to be another stone lighter and finally get into one or two of those fancy threads I bought with the proviso that 'One day I'll look good in these'.

Of course, for a fat bloke planning a weekend away, nothing is easy. When I was booking the tickets, I took the precaution of informing the airline's telephone help-desk that I was a fat bloke getting bigger and that I'd really like an outside seat – somewhere along the channel near the fourth row would be perfect. The call-centre, which presumably by the accents I encountered was in Bangalore, went into meltdown, with all sorts of middle managers running around in my earpiece screaming Bluetooth murder that under no circumstances was Channel 4 to be allowed anywhere near the plane.

When calm was restored, I was informed that, as a fat person, I was obliged to buy two seats for myself, and one for my wife. Trouble was, they couldn't guarantee them together, which was bloody odd, to say the least, and although I was booking an extra seat, I was told I could have a luggage allowance for only one person. So I hung up, went online, and booked a seat for a skinny bloke and one for his missus. Let the bastard who'll be sitting beside us worry that there's no room on his side of the seat. Like, what's the airline going to do: say I'm overweight and can't fly? I doubt it. And anyway, what airline carries a weighing scales to judge who is overweight and who isn't? So there you have it. The goal is set, and I'm four weeks away from a serious achievement. As Brutus might have said: 'O Julius Caesar, thou art mighty yet. Thy spirit will walk abroad and turn our swords of fat in our own proper entrails.'

Ten weeks ago, after many years of hardship and unease with my body, weight and eating habits, I made the radical decision to go on an all-out diet, with the intention of losing a few barbells around my stomach, to wear clothes that compliment the body instead of hide it, and to live a healthier and more all-encompassing life. Now, while I'm down about a stone and one and a quarter inches in trouser waist, and happy that I'm not lugging a small suitcase around with me everywhere I go, I do feel that I should be doing better.

My greatest difficulties have been psychological. No sooner had I made the decision to swap the belly for the ironing board than the securocrats who run my body were dashing around in my head screaming soliloquies, calling it a conspiracy and sending a clear message to my brain: 'Not on our watch, you won't.' Voices in your head, you say? OK, so it's a fat-bloke phenomenon. And how do these voices get their message across? Well, subtly really, playing me at the game I'm trying to play them at.

I can best describe it as mind games or, to be brutally honest, old-fashioned diabolical lying. When I decided I was going on a diet, I tricked my body, mind and self into believing that I wasn't really going on a diet at all – merely duck-walking a longer journey to the food mountain. Or, as the voices in my head would have it, finding a slower way to mega-obesity. So I put it about that, with a little window dressing, the pretence of taking a bit or two of veg, the odd soup on the side, and the occasional walk, everyone would think I'm the best fat bloke ever, and sure amn't I the great fella Francie, the Butcher Boy, for thinking it, so to speak. Well, as anyone who ever watched the George Sander classic *Village of the Damned* will know, it's not so easy keeping up in your mind a pretence behind a poorly built wall, especially with the id, ego and superego screaming at you in their bottle-blond wigs that they are going to pull it down brick by brick.

Of course, the three Freudian amigos knew something was up. No sooner had I put away the last morsel of Christmas pudding and everything else, literally as well as metaphorically, than the little gurriers had gathered restlessly around the cerebral hemisphere's water cooler gossiping about the secret messages that were been carried between my dietary advisors and my gut. Having tricked them into thinking I was on a diet, I was about to suffer a backlash. However, like any good liar – frantically keeping pace with the Pacman of deceit doing somersaults on the best Ferris wheel ever tied into complementary offshoots of DNA molecular geometry which jump in and out of the elevator like eager bellhops – I knew that tying my lie to a modicum of truth would save the day. This truth being that, yes, I wasn't going to forsake fast food forever, merely suggesting 'Let's give it up for a few days', knowing that after a few days my eating habits would be on a more even kilter and I wouldn't need to overeat. This argument luckily saved the day, and a diet was born.

Over the last ten weeks, while falling at least three times off the dietary cross, the three Freudian amigos continue to trouble and forsake me, particularly in my hour of greatest need. And of course I'm still lying to myself, hoodwinking an extra walk out of the old legs, or forsaking doughnuts for salads. Now, when I get an urge to have fast food, I tell the boyos, particularly the hedonistic id, who has always been the hardest to control in these circumstances: 'Yes, let's have some chips and burgers, but let's go for a walk or have a bowl of soup first.' Happy with a détente of sorts, and a quick jog around the block – or two ladles of homemade carrot soup – later, I and the rest of me is too full or tired to want anything else. It seems like a pain in the ass, but hey, it works for me.

And to be fair to my psyche, department policy is now firmly in favour of weight loss, proper diet and proportionality. The mindset, no longer the harbinger of snack boxes and midnight feasts, is now in training for the marathon, holding on to a slim chance that the body will actually run one. It also spends more shopping time in the vegetable aisles and hasn't been to biscuit-land for weeks. It might not be everyone's idea of a diet, but it's One Irishman's Diet.

Entering the second half of March, I was keen to get stuck in to a bit of serious exercise. Nothing life-threatening, you understand, but definitely something that would allow my body to breathe a little more, while losing a couple of extra pounds in the process. Not that my jogging experience hadn't made me wary. I was definitely reluctant to jog anywhere, with or without underpants or an emergency bandage of petroleum jelly. And I was definitely reluctant to go out at any hour of the day or night in a silly ill-fitting tracksuit. It's the fat jogger's paradox. Go out in the middle of the day and people will laugh at you, and every fourth car-owner thinks it's funny to honk his horn. And that's before you attract the bus-passengers, who wave at you as if you're doing it for charity, or you're some poor unfortunate who needs encouragement. What do you think we are, fairground attractions?

Night jogging is worse. Go out in the middle of the night dressed like a camouflaged elephant, and onlookers, taxi men and milkmen are likely to report you for suspicious behaviour. Do it yourself. Dress up like Humpty Dumpty and go out for a jog at two o'clock in the morning and try explaining to your local community policeman that 'Yes, I realise it's a mad time to be exercising. And, no matter how stupid it looks, yes, I do have a complex about other people seeing me in the daylight going for a jog. And no, I haven't been drinking.'

Of course, a fat bloke out jogging, wearing a hat to keep him warm in the middle of the night, is as guilty as a confession. Try telling a guard past the witching hour that the only reason you're wearing a head-warmer is because it's cold. Like, do I look as if I've modelled myself on Jack 'the Hat' McVitie? Like, how many fat robbers do you know who wear ridiculous-looking hats that barely cover their ears, never mind their mugs? And do you really think cat burglars use Friar Tuck cast-offs as a disguise? Besides, if I were to rob a bank in the middle of the night, I'd need a M1 Abrams main battle tank to make a hole big enough for me to fit through the bank's walls, and then have the wherewithal to carry the loot home while disposing of an armoured vehicle – that would be some *Dog Day After-midnight*, right? Quentin Tarantino isn't famous for *Reservoir Elephants* for no good reason, you know.

This wasn't the only thing putting me off jogging. The thought of all that pounding on ugly grey concrete also seemed too much to bear, all 17 – or is it 18? – stone of me (I've asked the wife to hide the weighing scales) beating down over my flabby knees and bulging ankles.

So what did I do? Well, I took up gardening. And not just any old gardening. No, I got myself an allotment, and a bloody big one to boot. So, what do I know about gardening? Well, let's put it this way, Monty Don isn't going to be worrying himself into a garden shed – or even Diamuid Gavin, who sounds peculiarly like Mary O'Rourke, come to think of it. But neither am I a complete gardening fool either. Apparently, it's in the genes: the old fellow thinks he's a bit handy with the green fingers. Anyway, in mid-March my delectable patch resembles a weed-graveyard, with the early frosts killing what little weed growth I have already.

Of course, any new hobby for me involves money, and I'm not one to take anything second-hand. So, early Saturday morning I raid the local gardening centre – with the wife in tow – and stock up on shovels, spades, compost, bulbs and plenty of seed. A pair of old boots, leggings from an old black tracksuit, and a long, free-flowing, multicoloured jumper later, I'm out in the wilds of the allotment standing on my shiny new shovel, like some mad super veg-patch Demis Roussos. And as gardening athletes will tell you, getting out there is the hardest part. Making that fateful decision to be a part of nature, reaching out for your green soul and foraging as God intended it, mucking it about under that little tent of blue, is sheer bliss, and definitely inspiring.

That is, until it suddenly dawns on you that gardening is a fancy word for digging and that, being the greedy bugger I am, it's going to take me weeks to dig my allotted patch. But hey, it's springtime, and the neighbours are all out around the square, with their English-country-garden straw hats, Christmas green sweaters and weathered tweeds. It's all jolly good fun standing there, the foot comatose on the shovel, waiting for someone to say it's OK to down tools and go home. However, this doesn't happen, and I'm forced to do a bit of work. And, by jaysus, it's hard work. The weeds, whom I can hear whispering to themselves 'Who the fuck's the new guy?', have been congealed in the undergrowth for the last ten years and are loath to leave their squat, embedded as they are. Stubborn, obstinate, and relishing a fight, they refuse to leave on the first tug. Or the second. Or even the third. I get a little more aggressive and start attacking the bastards with a vengeance. It's the Texas Chainsaw Massacre for weeds. Aaaaaaaagh! A neighbour comes over and politely asks me to pipe down, that my screeching is apparently frightening the children. I tell him I'm only joking. He looks at me as if I'm not only some sort of deranged fat bloke, but a Muppet to boot. 'And another thing, do you not have a pair of trousers big enough to hide the crack in your arse when you bend down? It's rather disgusting, actually.'

Anger aside, I want to pick up my tools and tunnel, not run or walk, back to my house, and hide my arse, face and shovels for eternity. However, before I have time to do anything, my neighbour offers some helpful encouragement: a bit of détente, you might say. 'Would you like to use the Rotavator we have down the other end? It's on hire for the weekend, and you can borrow it if you like?' I decline, begrudgingly. Could do with the exercise, I tell him. Moments later, I'm regretting it. Impulsive, you could say. Turn down help too easily. And, of course, once you've turned down help, particularly in the circumstances in which it was offered, it's very hard to go and say, 'I'm sorry, I am a stupid ungracious thoughtless Muppet, and I've just made a terrible impetuous mistake, and yes, I'd love to use your poxy Rotavator.'

Twenty minutes later, while I'm getting stuck into the obstinate ground, my wife turns up to give me moral support. Support-your-local-fat-bloke sort of thing. She's also here to do a bit of her own gardening. I decide it's best not to mention the offer of the Rotavator, although I'm sure she can hear the racket they're making down at the end of the field. And of course, she's come prepared. Gloves, cloths, water (there are camels who carry less water than my wife), handy forks, secateurs, scissors, multiple tie-racks, bamboo poles, netting, trowels, and a miserable-looking pole of unhappiness that goes by the name of a hoe.

A hoe, you say? That's what I said. A hoe? Wasn't that what all those down-at-heel Chinese farmer-types carried in that 1970s television series *Kung Fu*? Those poor unfortunates on the lowest rung of the American dream, working in mines, building the Iron Horse, or carrying the gold-diggers' mules and handle-less frying pans, slowly building California's Chinatown, unable to go to the post office or the drugstore without some unshaven ex-pillar of the local jail kicking ten shades of shite out of them. That is, until Kwai Chang Caine (David Carradine) arrived.

Sadly, in my present circumstances, it's unlikely that somebody is going to creep up on me on rice paper and surreptitiously dig the allotment for me. So, 'Sorry love,' I titter in a manly sort of way, 'I won't be using one of those.' If it wasn't good enough for Caine, it won't be good enough for me.

Of course, the story of the hoe goes a little deeper. Earlier in the weekend, I had laughed at my wife when she'd bought the hoe in the gardening centre when I was shelling out on a similar apparatus that could best be described as the thinnest gardening fork you could ever find, the head just about big enough to eat your dinner with if you were 10 foot 6 tall, with long arms and a big mouth.

Minutes later, while I'm struggling to dislodge a line of weeds with my useless beanpole fork, my wife is making easy progress digging below the surface weed line and ripping out the invaders in one easy motion. I'm immediately smitten; no, envious. I want to sidle up to her and say, 'Master, forgive me, for I have failed. And, now that you mention it, could I borrow the hoe?' Only for her to say: 'You have failed no one, Grasshopper, only your ambition.' But that doesn't happen, and when I just ask if I can borrow the hoe, she says 'No.' No? 'Yes, no.' And it's final. Apparently, the difference of opinion – she called it an 'episode' – in the gardening centre touched a nerve, the facts of which I've probably been a little more succinct about than I should have been. So, without waiting to ask twice, I'm in the car, up the road, into the garden centre, circumnavigating the 'Jesus, Phyllis, there's a rush on the hoes, that's two in four years', paid, bought, 'No, love, I don't need a bag', and back in the allotment before you can say 'Get your mucky boots off the rice paper'.

Hoe, hoe, hoe, it's off to work we go, and before long I'm at least two of the Seven Dwarfs – Grumpy and Sleepy – with the premonition that by the middle of summer I'll also be Sneezy, given my hay-fever malignancy. All I'm missing is the gnome-like hat and the beard down to my feet.

Two hours into my life as a gentleman farmer, I have suddenly developed an obsessional hatred of the dandelion family. As a matter of course, I want to murder all things yellow. It's like coming into my Herod phase: I feel that if I kill every dandelion under two years old, I'll be king forever in my allotment. That's before I even come to grips with the daddy of the dandelion menace, the flying jinny-joes – those little grey-white bits of fluff that children often blow while making a wish. By mid-afternoon, when I've finally put the yellow bastards to bed, a bit of a wind has kicked up, and the jinny-joes – or dandelion clocks, to give them their proper name – are flying around my patch like an out-of-season Santa Claus on a jolly, dropping Little Boy seeds where my potatoes and vegetables were promised.

Back-breaking as the work is, though, I seem to be getting somewhere, both with my allotment and with my need for physical exercise, albeit slowly. And it is slow, really slow. Knackeringly slow, even, although I persevered when I felt that the weight was falling off me. So much so that every two hours I had to go indoors to change my extra-extra-extra large T-shirts – which not surprisingly are pink and orange. Try getting fat clothes in colours that don't make you out to be a melon, a grapefruit or a body double for General Lee in *The Dukes of Hazzard*: it's practically impossible. On the way in to change one of my pink T-shirts, our postman, unusually delivering on a Saturday, spots me from about a hundred yards down the road, and let's rip so as all the neighbours can hear him: 'Fair play to you. It takes a real man to wear a pink T-shirt.' From behind lamp-posts, car bonnets, children's prams and windows, heads pop out to clarify that the fat bloke in the pink T-shirt is indeed their neighbour. Jesus, the embarrassment.

By dinner time, I've gone through all my fruity extra-extra-extra-large T-shirts, and I'm finally down to the large Calvin Klein T-shirt I bought in America about six years ago – a T-shirt that's so big you could hide an elephant in it. Sweltering in the early-spring heat, the salt in my system has gathered on my arms and brow, like 'Charlie' lined up for a nose inspection. In between a yard of hoeing here and half a yard of subsequent digging there, I've borrowed most of the camel's water, an arrangement that caused a bit of friction. People who tend to bring their own water on picnics with them are the type of people who never want to share. Just because you forgot your refreshments doesn't mean they can run the Little Red Hen parable over me. No, sir.

APRIL

MINI-BREAK TO BORDEAUX AND THE MECHANICS, HISTORY AND PSYCHOLOGY OF A CHIP OBSESSION

Bordeaux was supposed to be a New Year incentive to lose weight, although I had bought the tickets on Christmas Eve, ostensibly as a Christmas present for my wife. A stocking-filler, you understand, and a target for myself to get in shape, drop a few pounds, and fit into the multitude of clothes that waited in the wardrobe like young lovers under Clerys' clock for their first date. But, by April, and the weekend of the short-break holiday, the weighing scales (once it arrived back from absentia) wasn't showing any major sign of improvement. I was still hovering around 17 and a half stone, and still trying in vain to slide out of my 41-inch waistline. With the high-blood-pressure thermostat on a panic setting doing loop-the-loop, this necessitated an emergency shopping trip to supplement my wardrobe. I had nothing to wear. Zilch. Zero. Ne'er a stitch. And the combination of cantankerous, trouser-tight and shirt-busting husband with an excited holiday-minded wife going on a short break is one of those pressure sores that can lead to divorce.

I really thought I'd done much better. I seemed a lot healthier, was certainly getting a proper night's sleep, and felt more comfortable in my clothes; these, of course, being my winter attire. Temperatures in Bordeaux in mid-April can reach the mid-twenties centigrade, but I had enough long-armed jumpers, woollen socks, big-faced shoes and bulging tracksuits for any amount of snow, rain, sleet or pessimistic predictions from a plethora of climate-warming Green Party party-poopers who might feel compelled to spell out the greenhouse scenario that's sure to end in an Ice Age Armageddon. Sadly, time was the real issue, with even the most sober weather forecasters prophesying more heat before the great forces in our universe push the buttons on the *fin de siècle* chill. So, unless the earth started accelerating rapidly around the sun – travelling three hundred years over a weekend – or if every single Chinese on the planet went out and bought four fridges each and then decided simultaneously to release every smidgen of coiled-up CFC into the ozone layer over a three-day period, I was going to be the proverbial snowman, if there is such a thing, dressed for exile in a desert.

And it's not as though I haven't had this problem before. There was the time on the mid-term break to the Canaries when, once again laden down with the weight penalty, I was absolutely miserable, not least with the problem that developed with my feet. Most people planning a sun holiday remember to pack sun-tan lotions, after-sun, mosquito treatments, paracetamol and anti-histamines. Some people even bring medicine chests. And while we can all be neurotic about caring for our skin, our teeth, our eyes, our nose and even our hangovers, we rarely protect our feet.

I used to think that way too, but that was before the Fuerteventura episode. On the third day of our holiday, my wife and I booked a trip on a catamaran. Big mistake. Like most of these money-sucking adventure enterprises, there were rules, and I hate rules, particularly if they are pointless or over-officious, or if, on the morning we're hooking up with all the other happy holiday-campers, my shorts and T-shirts are so tight around my body that I feel I'm in bondage to the whole damn world. Anyway, the rule on this treble-hulled, reinforced-fibreglass monstrosity was simple: passengers weren't allowed on board wearing shoes or socks. Worse still, and a blatant contradiction to my mind, the crew were exempt from this rule.

Initially, I was having none of it. I was feeling awkward. I wanted to ask for our money back, or to start a Fletcher Christian-style mutiny among my fellow holiday-makers, or, if that didn't work, maybe try a little subtle blackmail, where I'd address the passengers with something akin to: 'Do you all mind me wearing no sandals, bearing in mind that I have a rather large verruca.' Prophetic words, indeed. My wife felt that I was over-reacting and that maybe the crew knew best, and, of course, she really didn't want another scene. Another scene? Well, yes, there were mitigating circumstances. I had already objected to the ship's resident David Bailey taking my photograph, and his buddy, the Pedro Almodóvar of the Canaries, videoing my every movement under the pretence that we were all friends and it was a lovely day, when I knew they were running the old 'Do you want to buy a video or photograph?' trick. So, to avoid the ignominy of a third 'misunderstanding', I shut up, with a St Peter-like denial that left my feet with a rather large cross to bear.

Two weeks later, that cross arrived, at probably the same moment as Mr and Mrs 'Well we've no problem taking off our shoes' were receiving (if they were lucky) their catamaran videos and happy snapshots. Having a little discomfort walking (a burning sensation), I checked my feet. Just below the big toe on my left foot, I noticed a nice juicy verruca. How big was it? Well, you could just about write 'Made in Fuert . . . ' across the middle. And so began the long process of eradication, with the usual stages of denial, acceptance and treatment.

Anyway, getting back to the trip to Bordeaux. Trousers and shirts – well, there was the perennial problem. For anyone with a weight sentence living in a bubble, everyday problems don't really exist until you knock on the door of 'thin world'. As I've said earlier, once you expose yourself in any shape or form, out from beneath the friendly bushels or grassy knoll – where any fat person could have shot Kennedy and got away with it (example: Lee Harvey Oswald was thin, Jack Ruby wasn't) – the problems gallop over the prairie like Custer leading the 7th Cavalry into the Battle of the Little Big Horn, obviously named for a gluttonous schizophrenic, if judicious, Native American whose real name was Tepee Sitting-Couch Potato-Bull and a senior partner in Sioux, Sioux and More Sioux – who wanted to be thin. And, right in the thick of the action, the wife starts butting in and offering her oar's-worth: 'I thought you said you were going to lose weight' or 'I told you not to eat those chips. Did you listen to me? No, no, no'. The pressure points in your veins go into spasm, confused about whether now is a good time to give you a heart attack or the incentive to learn the bloody lesson. Lost – well, you wish you were. But no, the wife ratchets up the anxiety, going over all your previous most shameful habits and giving you the angry-matron sermon and gambling with your patience threshold. You know a row is about to kick off.

You offer mitigating circumstances. Three months into a diet of sorts, with a waistband still clocking up the mileage on its regular trip around the globe-girth, and my inner organs doing twelve rounds with the ghost of Ali, I still thought I'd made some progress. I'm no longer a fat 42-inch waster (or should that be 'waister'), my belly cliff hanging over the precipice, hiding my toes below. And, yes, my stomach has definitely slowed down on the day trips and is a little trimmer, a step back from the breach, from that thin line across my Rubicon, dividing one half of my body from the other. And, like its more illustrious Roman original – the Rubicon, I mean – I feel that no fat Generalissimo lying under siege in my lower gut will feel brave enough to cross the line between insurrection and the Republic of Me. If I had been around in Roman times, that noble biographer Suetonius, to paraphrase JC – no, not that JC, Julius Caesar – would have mistaken me for Pompey the Great and said of me that 'This fat man knows how to win a war'; or maybe a modern-day dictator or general like Lucius Cornelius Sulla might have commented of me as Sulla pass-remarked on Julius Caesar: 'Beware the boy with the loose clothes.' Loose clothes, now there's a dream. Waffle, I'm told. It's all waffle. The mutterings of a fool. As the wife cuts me down to size, I'm left to face realities.

I've also had my spring appointment at the liver clinic. Every time I go to the clinic, I follow the same procedure, and it's straight out of a Neil Simon play. I arrive, hand over my appointment card to the secretary, who updates my details – or says she does, even though there is generally nothing to update. Then she tells me to go downstairs to a weighing room, where a nurse weighs me on an electronic scales. The nurse writes my weight on a piece of paper – I'm obviously not bright enough to be asked to trust it to memory – and I then go upstairs again into the waiting room next door to the secretary's office, where, if I've been careful enough to make an early appointment, I'm the only person there. I have occasionally forgotten to do this and have found myself waiting to be seen for a 2 PM appointment, three hours later. Anyway, however long I've been waiting, the secretary will wake me from my slumber and tell me to go up the stairs to a particular room, where a doctor will give me a good talking to on the reasons why I've got a fatty liver, mention the benefits of a proper diet and regular exercise, and then offer to book me a session with a dietician, which I respectfully decline. 'It's in my head, doc,' I protest. 'Psychological-like, do you know what I mean? And anyway, I eat all the right foods. It's just that I tend to eat all the wrong ones with them.' Then we shake hands and promise to see each other again in six months' time. I then go back down the stairs, ask the secretary for the earliest appointment six months later, and the cycle begins again.

Anyway, the spring appointment is a failure. I'm still not tuned into the dangers of fatty liver. His second opinion, for which I was grateful, offered the diagnosis that I wasn't an alcoholic but that I had a liver problem. Fatty liver, which carries the calling card *steatorrhoeic hepatosis* or *steatosis hepatitis*, is apparently a reversible condition where large vacuoles of triglyceride fat accumulate in the liver cells of people who drink too much or who suffer from obesity. I'm in the latter category, and this time the specialist in the liver clinic sends me for a glucose-tolerance test. This involves going down to the hospital and having your bloods taken. You're then asked to drink a bottle of Lucozade and sent to the waiting room for two hours, after which your bloods are taken again. Examining the effects of the Lucozade on the blood against the blood before the test determines whether you are a diabetic or on the way to becoming one. My result shows that, while I'm not borderline diabetic, I'm the borderline below. It's what you might call another failure.

*

And so the cycle begins for another year. The mad dash into town to secure clothing for the mid-term break: another three pairs of forty-two-inch trunk liners, two pairs of eighteen-inch shirts, a casual jacket to match everything and up another size in the jocks. Make sure to keep receipts in case, God forbid, I lose two stone over the French weekend or have the good fortune to get away with wearing one pair of trousers for the whole weekend, thus allowing me to bring everything back first thing Monday morning. Am I exaggerating? Not really, because although I was bringing my one faithful pair of trousers for casual wear and the dressy pair of slacks I use for the weddings and funerals, going to a region that produces really warm spring weather, I felt I needed something to blend in more, without catching the eye of the locals as the fat Irishman in the duffle.

With the exception of the jacket, I hadn't time to try anything on, mainly because, being in such a rush, my jockeys were soaking, having filled up with sweat that had dripped out of glands I didn't know existed, and resembled one of those magic sponges football trainers used to carry in their kitbags. Thus the wet sponge between my legs was now acting as an adhesive to my crotch. The thought of taking off my trousers to try on a new pair and exposing the soggy groin line in my nether regions to the air revolted me with the insinuation that, if I did it, who else was doing it? And am I putting on a pair of trousers that some other eighteen-stone mucky duck tried on before me? (With clothes this big, the identikit is always the same, and you can't get away from the conclusion that a fat bloke has tried on the clothes you're thinking about buying.) Better to buy the lot, try them on at home – where I could have a bath afterwards – and then bring back to the shop anything that didn't fit. With this bit of last-minute shopping, 'The job was oxo', as my Uncle Joe used to say.

Everything about getting from Dublin to Bordeaux on Aer Lingus was uneventful, from the rain on the way to the airport to the rain on the way to the hotel, save from a minor row with the Dublin taxi man – not on my time, buddy – who wanted to go his own way to Dublin Airport. Other than flying in over the big wide expanses of the Gironde estuary and the typically French white-stone architecture, you could have been, as far as the weather went, anywhere at home. Knowing that we were flying in relatively late in the afternoon, I put on my old trousers and shirt, so as not to wear out any of the threads that I had just bought. Traditionally, on the first days of such holidays, I also wear my oldest pair of jockeys, or those ones with the bullet-holes, leaving them wherever I find myself on that all-important first night. In recent times, I'm sure cleaning staff on Irish Ferries, Brittany Ferries and hotels in New York, Barcelona and Paris, to name a few, have discovered well-used Irish jocks in those tight little foot-pedal waste buckets that never open as easily as they're supposed to and lounge in bathroom corners more as a furniture accessory than as a serious Tombstone coffin for used jocks. Not that that usually puts me off. Wherever you're likely to find such a final resting place, my Gunfight at the OK Corral jockeys are likely to have been there before you. Not surprisingly, for this reason, I never open a foot-pedal bin of any description without using my foot, or, in extreme cases, without at least two pairs of rubber gloves.

Anyway, bused in from the airport – Aeroport de Bordeaux – the journey, in the late-afternoon rain, was at least cool enough for me to hide inconspicuously in my winter woollies. The wife, of course, was all summery and already in holiday mood, and no amount of fat-boy slimming or complaining was going to upset her. I, on the other hand, had made my bed – or should that be my over-thoughtful breakfasts, lunches, evening meals and over-fatty in-betweens – and no matter how much I dared deviate from my circumstances, I was going to have to sleep in it. And woe betide me if I said anything to the contrary.

So there we were, ensconced three floors up at Hotel Majestic on rue de Condé, a street immediately parallel to Cours 30 Juillet – which I obviously took not as a reference to the date England won the World Cup in 1966 or to the birth of Emily Brontë but as a nod to the July Revolution of 1830, the abdication of King Charles X and the whole shenanigans on the balcony of the city hall in Paris, where the old codger Lafayette gave Louis-Philippe, the Duc d'Orléans, the famous kiss and the return of the Tricolour that had been banned since Napoleon's political demise in 1815. Cours 30 Juillet is fairly near Bordeaux's main thoroughfare, which rambles down to Place de la Comédie, where, naturally, there's a theatre. The Grand Theatre, what the locals call an 'architectural masterpiece', was built in a neo-classical design by Victor Louis between 1773 and 1780, although I'm not sure if this means that it took him seven years to build it or that it was built during this period and that somebody forget to write down the date. You wouldn't have had that problem during the Terror a few years later, where if you didn't mark the important occasions, you could be assured of a visit from Madame la Guillotine herself. Nothing like a bit of fear to garnish results, I say. Although, whenever I'm in France, I prefer never to mention the Terror, just as you wouldn't mention World War II in Germany. Mind you, it's always a bit embarrassing for Irish people when it comes to these sorts of things. When most nations were at war sixty-odd years ago, we were having an Emergency. Who says victors write their own history – surely they meant neutrals.

The Grand Theatre – which I would have been able to see from our bedroom window if I had Spiderman's wrists, ability to swing on air, love of heights and a bit of web-gel – is a monster of a building with twelve Corinthian columns supporting an entablature (yeah, I don't know what it means either), on which stand twelve statues that represent the nine muses and three goddesses, Juno, Venus, and Minerva. Sitting in Room 12 of Hotel Majestic at twelve minutes past seven, and looking out at a deserted twelve-room office building 'à vendre' at € 12 million across the narrow street, I got an eerie feeling that the number twelve was pretty significant in these parts. The thought lasted a moment as my mind reacted to the word 'garnish' (a paragraph back) and pressed some internal buttons, alerting my stomach, eating disorder and sensory glands that it was dinner time in a foreign city and that one big fat-arsed Irishman should be thinking of food.

So out we went into the spring evening, which had perked up considerably since the afternoon but was still spitting rain on the other side of our umbrella. It had been nearly six hours since my last snack (bless me, Father, for these are my sins: a giant sandwich and a surreptitious packet of crisps) in Dublin. Internally, I felt that Times Square was calling me to dinner, its lights shining illumination and temptations at the heart of my obsessions. When the wife reads this, she will know that 'Yes, I was right, you did have a packet of crisps' and that 'Yes, the red marks on your gums are your over-zealous attempts at covering up your eating disorder with toothpaste'. Apparently, the ingredients in a tube of toothpaste aren't what they used to be, and cannot be guaranteed to wash away the ole Tayto or King, and yes, it doesn't matter how hard you brush.

After about an hour and a half of looking around for somewhere that fitted our appetites, we found a suitable restaurant. When I say 'suitable restaurant', what I really mean is an eatery that serves chips. Not that my wife is usually aware of this habitual procession, and the excuses of 'Nah, I'm not sure I could eat in a room where the décor's darker than the night', to 'Jesus, it's too bright in there', or 'No, I don't want fish', or 'It's too late for steak: it'll stick in my stomach all night'. So, while my wife runs her finger down the menu, eyeing the reasonably sensible *salade de chèvre chaude* or outrageously suggesting that 'seeing as it's late' – or presumably because we're monks on a busman's holiday and should take a vow of abstinence – 'we should probably only go for one course', I'm climbing the walls, going in the opposite direction, dismissing all the healthy options that have only got standing room beside my *pommes frites* obsession. I've had this chip obsession since I was a child. It's a bigger burden than the third secret of Fatima, and I don't care how long it took you wrestling with your conscience to tell us you were in the Hitler Youth.

When your mind can think only of chips, it doesn't matter where you are in the world – The Vatican, Rome, Bordeaux, Dublin – or whose fancy half-arsed banquet you're sitting at. When that call comes spiralling through the food-sensors to the controls in your head, there's only one way to order: 'I'll have the chips, please.' There hasn't been a restaurant, pub, diner or roadway food-shack I've gone anywhere in my life with my wife or otherwise where she hasn't said to me either a) compassionately, b) in anger, or c) with extreme anger: 'Don't order the chips.'

When I say 'or otherwise', I mean – and I'll discuss this more fully in later chapters – she's my conscience, half-woman/wife/lover sitting in front of me, half-voice in my head shouting: 'Don't order the chips.' Whether she's reading the menu at the same table as me or raiding my consciousness when she's not around, her little face, turned obtusely – and I use the word mathematically, for my wife's intellect is anything but slow – like a triangle trying to crawl sideways up a hill without the use of its arms, offering a softly, softly approach that's made up of manners, facial expressions and body language, which quickly gives way to an urgency after realising the diplomacy isn't working. 'Don't order the chips', she warns, her face back firmly on her shoulders, the angle receding away from the acute angle more into my face than out of it. It's an image that tends to stay with you, and may as well be living in the rented accommodation of my conscience. In many ways, she's more my conscience than my conscience itself.

In fact, I've thought of plenty of ways to order chips without my wife's – or my conscience's – consent. If I ever meet Magnus Magnusson in the great *Mastermind* in the sky, and he was ever to ask my specialist subject, I'd probably say: 'Ten thousand ways to order chips without the wife knowing.' Such devilish cunning has included adding chips to the order, on the pretence to my wife that I'm slipping to the toilet, and instead whispering to the waiter over the counter to 'Add an extra portion of chips to the order, but not so my wife will notice it', giving the impression that they come with the meal and that the restaurant either doesn't know the value of chips or is incredibly generous, and picking a fight with a waiter to the tune of 'No, I didn't order the chips when my wife went to powder her nose, smart-arse.' I even once convinced my wife that fast-food chains offer complimentary chips if you buy two burgers, on the financial nous that all the profit is in the meat.

Psychologically, since I went through Piaget's later stages of pre-operation, and certainly well before I mastered his M&M trick for the first time, I have probably thought about chips at least once a day, every day of my life. Even when I'm not having chips, I'm thinking of having them the following day. Whether it's in bed or in the bath, my mind often slides into a chip van or chip shop. Like all obsessions, this one began at home, back in the years when my mother's wooden spoon was a secret weapon. Traditionally, my mother used to make chips on a Friday – the usual Catholic Ireland 1970s ritual serving with fish. I'd say I had home-made chips every Friday of my life until somewhere in my low teens. My mother decided that Wednesday would be a good day to have chips as well, adding an extra day's plate of fish to the menu. It was almost as if, unconsciously, she was aware that there was some great malignancy in the chips and that the fish, with its religious connotations, was capable of cleansing the sin before it even had time to arrive in some judge's basket in heaven. Now, that's not to say that my mother was a bad mother. In fact, at the time, I thought she was great, and ahead of her time. I still do. And although our family never did vox pops, to the tune of 'Do you enjoy having chips Wednesdays and Fridays?', I can't remember any dissent or family referenda on having my mother burned at the stake or the Spanish Inquisition arriving to ask her if Christ owned his own chip pan? Obviously, at the time, every member of the clan was on the same diet and, from what I can tell, I'm probably the only one scourged with the obsession, although it's not a condition I've canvassed, spoken widely about or made overtures to the family elders about over the years. And anyway, it's not like my family are going anywhere in the next number of years. I could wait another forty or fifty years for their take on what seems like a hidden family secret. It's not as though my father is likely to be standing on top of some formidable rock-face in the Dublin mountains looking into an abyss and writing the family epitaph without mentioning my chip obsession to the melody of 'I Chingachgook O'Doherty have lived to see the last warrior of the wise race of the O'Doherty Mohicans'.

Before I lose track of the chip story, I must remind myself that the only other day I had home-made chips was on regular Thursday visits to my Granny Doherty's in Cabra when I was small. She made the most magnificent chips. If ever there was a Queen of Chips, it was Granny Doherty. Now, that's not to say that my mother's chips weren't good. They were very good. It was just – and I'm not one to harp on about percentages – that the mother's chips were only 80 percent as good as Granny Doherty's. It was only after persistent 'Ma, why can't you make chips like Granny Doherty' that my mother let me in on one of the family's chip secrets, when she, you could say rather scurrilously, pointed out that Granny Doherty's secret ingredient was tripe, what you might call a poor man's Crisp-n-Dry substitute. 'Yes, Paul,' she said, pointing at the slime on the lower reaches of the butcher's shelf the following day. 'That white slithery piece there at the front – that's the O'Doherty family's secret ingredient.' While those were the days long before mad-cow disease rode into town with a science book under its arm, offal, edible or otherwise, wasn't exactly something I could stomach, to use a bad pun, especially since it lay there like some bloated upside-down wheelbarrow. Jesus, I said to myself, my Granny's been serving me that – 'offal', you say – 'made from the stomach of God knows how many Friesians/Holsteins and other furry animals'.

My Granny Doherty died when I was twelve, by which time, possibly, my only regret was not asking her did she ever use beef tripe – which is typically made from the first three of any cow's four stomachs. Or did she ever remember using the rumen flattish eiderdown-smooth tripe or the reticulum honeycomb and pockety type (I can only imagine where that one gets its name from) or what some Christians call the omasum or bible-leaf variety. Either way, I've never eaten tripe since, knowingly, on or off my chips, and can only add in conclusion to the Granny Doherty story that if tripe was the only grease ever used in chip-making, I would have buried my obsession years ago. Years later, I mentioned this story to my mother. 'Tripe?' says she. 'I never said that. Sure who in their right mind ever used tripe to make chips? You couldn't make chips with tripe even if you wanted to – you're probably thinking of dripping.' 'Dripping? No, no,' says I, 'do you not remember the conversation in the butchers when I was ten?' 'No I don't. That's all in your imagination, and don't be telling anybody otherwise.' To this day, I'm still waiting for her to put me wise, and admit to a conversation that she claims never took place.

Anyway, to recap, I've only ever had home-made chips on Wednesdays, Thursdays and Fridays. That is except for that one occasion on a Sunday when my mother was in hospital having my younger sister, and my father, a lost soul in the kitchen, decided to treat me and my younger brother to overcooked chips. I think my mother still harbours nightmares of denial that any of her children were ever served chips on the Sabbath, even if it wasn't on her watch. Other than that, I only ever had chips (and anyway, they weren't home-made) when I was younger if my mother and father brought them home on the way back from the pub on a weekend night – which, to be fair, wasn't very often.

As time went by, this obsession grew. (I'm not sure why I haven't referred to it as an addiction yet. I constantly refer to my problem as an obsession, but that's a sidestep from diagnosing its real identity: an addiction, what you might call the real elephant in the room. What's obsessional is easily ignored by the chattering classes, including the ones in my own head, as 'just one of those things', something to ignore and 'Sure, it'll probably go away'. Mention addiction, and it's the Premier League. Knocking out Darlington in the second round of the Johnstone's Paint Trophy suddenly becomes front-page news, as if you've mentioned Chelsea, astronomical ticket prices or whether John Terry should be on £120,000 a week. The scrutiny police come staring and enlarged, with their square-shaped heads, through the spyhole in your mind's eye. You're dragged away for questioning to some Kafkaesque castle, where the square-heads want to know how you never mentioned you had an addiction and how you, Gregor Samsa, just managed to wake up one morning having inexplicably metamorphosed your obsession into a full-blown addiction. What? What?)

Anyway . . . the problem was that chips twice or three times a week wasn't enough to feed my growing fixation on the humble potato dunked in oil. And so, every time my mother went out to the meetings she attended in the evenings – she was a serial meeting-goer when we were young – which seemed to coincide with nights when my father was at work, and when my younger brother and sister were also long in bed, I'd serve up chips for myself. And I'm not talking a plate here or there; I'm talking mega-food.

At the time, I remember being fussy about how I even made the bloody things. I probably convinced myself that I was even a bit of a gourmet. The first couple of batches had to be just about cooked, with the fluffy potato beginning to turn a slightly yellowy golden colour, followed by a couple of smaller consignments allowed to oil up a little longer, concluding with the last batch, which always had to be much crisper and crunchier than its predecessors, on what you might call the rare side of burnt. And, although it was verboten in our house to make chips out of new potatoes, in the same way that it was forbidden to make toast with fresh bread – how times have changed – I particularly liked chips made from the newest of new potatoes, especially if they were floury. At the time, I didn't know it, but King Edwards or Maris Pipers were my favourites. It's worth noting that in those days, making chips with what amounted to soapy or watery potatoes (I hated watery vegetables) was also an occasional cure for my chip obsession, where there was no chance of the chips crisping up and hiding the floury goodness inside. Luckily, using soapy potatoes was an affliction that I rarely came across; not like today, where finding good potatoes is like trying to ram the arse of a camel through the eye of a needle. Although, if the worldwide obesity problem is to be believed, it's going to to be a hell of a lot easier for a rich man to get into heaven than it is to get anyone (particularly if we all continue to grow fatter) through the eye of an needle.

Of course, making chips when my parents weren't around wasn't done with their blessing. So, since I've been making chips since I was very young, this required a considerable amount of planning and subterfuge. According to the stories doing the rounds in those days, in the years before kids went to school to become crime-scene investigators, every second house burnt down because the chip pan hadn't been properly supervised. It was my parents' standard warning when they occasionally discovered my extra-curricular eating habits: 'Don't put on the chip pan when we're not here. The house will catch fire and we'll all have to live on the side of the road.' Which, to be fair to my parents, wasn't a threat that we were going to join the travelling community – as if membership was something you subscribed to by paying the church collection. They were well aware that it wasn't part of our tradition to travel. And you couldn't very well pull up with no caravan and say to the elders of the travelling community, 'How's it going? Our house burned down because little Paulie used the chip pan when he wasn't supposed to, so we're joining yeh.' 'You are like fuck', they'd have told us. 'Like, do you think we have spare road-sites to give to anybody. Fuck off back to the settled community before we set the dogs on yeh.' (My parents' other standard warning was that I was, upon pain of death, never to swim in the canal because I might get polio, and 'Did I want to end up in a wheelchair?' This despite my continued assurances that I knew no one who went swimming in the canal in a wheelchair.)

Whatever the true story, it gave the startling impression that everybody seemed to be living or dying of chips in Ireland, or that they were mind-numbingly careless in the kitchen, or that every second eejit was buying a dodgy chip pan from Flash Harry types.

Doing a bit of my own research, I quickly realised that chip shops never burnt down, suggesting that, whatever the Italians were doing, they were at least doing it right. This was around the time when the second food-bearing wave of the Italian diaspora arrived in Ireland, not to sell us pizza or pasta, as you'd expect, but to sell us fish and chips, something you couldn't get in their own country – not that that was a problem. In later years, it would be the demonic snack box – with, of course, the two breasts of chicken – that would vie with my home-made chips as the experience of choice when I would stop off from the daily routine to beef up on breaded chicken in a sea of chips. Anyway, the advice from the local fire officers was that most of the fires in people's kitchens were caused by idiots trying to move their blazing chip pans off their cookers and out into their back gardens. It was suggested that throwing a wet teacloth (it didn't say from what distance or with how much ferocity) over the burning chip pan was a much better solution. Consequently, in the days before the arrival of deep-fat fryers, I always had three wet teacloths on standby, just in case. So much so that my mother was forever complaining that there wasn't a dry cloth in the house. Now she knows why.

Trying to deceive my parents that I wasn't making chips every time they turned their backs was like trying to pull the wool over the combined awareness of McMillan and Wife, The Hardy Boys and Nancy Drew's Maw and Paw. Firstly, there were the raw materials: electricity, chip pan, oil and potatoes. Electricity wouldn't be something most people would think of on *Celebrity Family Fortunes* if the question was 'In answer to our survey, what did people say were the key ingredients you'd need to hide if you wanted to outwit a seven-year-old who had a chip obsession and who couldn't stop making chips every time your back was turned?' But it was something my mother thought of every time she went out. In her wisdom, she often unplugged the cooker, thinking, well, if he switches on the cooker and nothing happens, little Paul will think that the man from the Leco board is on holidays or playing hide-and-seek with Hansel and Gretel. No, sir, not to my senses, he wasn't. He was generally the bloke who spent the 1970s on strike with his mates while we sat in bloody darkness listening to the radio and trying to figure out if Clondalkin, where we lived, was in Zone A or Zone B. So, if the electricity didn't work, and every other appliance in the house was plodding along just fine, well obviously the cooker's not plugged in. Job fixed, and on we go.

The chip pan was a more awkward item to replace. Frequently, I knew when my mother was going out long before she'd tell anyone, because the chip pan would go missing. Where did she hide it? Well, I would search everywhere, and mostly to no avail. Upstairs, downstairs, even out in the shed. I suspect she hid it in my father's car, for, as Sherlock Holmes says, if you rule out everywhere that's logical, it can only be in the place that's left – which was invariably the car. Holmes should have known, having his own addiction – cocaine. She once hid the chip pan in a four-stone bag of potatoes, thinking, well, he'll probably go looking for the chip pan first (and not the potatoes), and if he can't find it, he'll of course never think to look first in the sack of potatoes. Reverse psychology. And he'll just go back to proving Pythagoras's Theorem wrong, or trying to figure out why Michael Collins didn't blow Éamon de Valera away first when he had the chance. Wrong. If I couldn't find the chip pan, I improvised. Other pots and pans, while not ideal – the pots burned too easily, and the pans were too shallow – were scattered around the kitchen and only inviting me with shouts of 'Me, Me, Me'. By the time the deep-fat fryer had superseded the chip pan, hiding the larger electrical appliance was a lot more difficult for the mother, although for a time she would hide the basket – as if that would work.

Oil was always a problem. Easier to hide than the pan itself, it was also more difficult to find. It was the one item that regularly stumped me. The oil crisis in the 1970s, for me, didn't mean long queues outside petrol stations or wondering if the whole world was going to come to one giant full stop. It was the emergency to end all emergencies: how was I to get oil to cook my favourite chips? Hiding the oil became de rigueur in our house. It was something that was never left out unless it was Wednesday or Friday. On other days, it may as well have been renditioned through Shannon in an orange jumpsuit for all I was aware. It didn't exist. And without it, I couldn't make chips. I did try other options, such as Frytex and butter, but the taste wasn't the same, and I ended up using far more than I needed, which defeated the purpose of hiding my over-eating and brought the Homeland Security Food Police down on me before I could say 'That's not a real wooden spoon'.

Potatoes, strangely enough, were almost never hidden, and were therefore the easiest of the ingredients to find. We always had potatoes in the house, because they were the staple component of the family's diet. If the bag of potatoes was not standing up straight, my mother knew that it was time to order another four-stone bag from one of the vegetable men, who arrived most Fridays, selling his spuds and seasonal veggies. Her strategy was simple. She never hid the potatoes unless she had plans to go out at the end of the week at a time when I might be tempted to make chips, in which case she was more likely to allow stocks to run down. Consequently, when potatoes were in abundance, I would hide what I considered to be a reasonable amount in case of emergencies, for the unexpected announcement of 'Paul, I'm going out for an hour or two: don't make chips'. 'Paul, don't make chips' became a form of greeting between my mother and me, although

I was acutely aware that she smarmily uttered it only when she knew, or thought she knew, that there wasn't an earthly chance I was going to make chips when she was out. As time went by, I also tried to put away as much oil as I could for such sudden disclosures.

I once tried hiding the spuds in the ground in the back yard, only for my father to find them and come running into the house proclaiming a miracle. 'Jesus, I'm after finding new potatoes in the ground, spot-perfect, and this not yet the end of February.'

Eating the blessed chips was easy, if a little tiring. Once they had all been devoured, it was time to clean up the evidence, knowing full well that my parents wouldn't be away all night and that speed was of the essence. Obviously, not having had any IRA experience of cleaning a crime scene, I had to use all my instincts to evade detection by getting rid of the circumstantial evidence. Cleaning up was run-of-the-mill. Two plates, a knife and fork, and a squirt of Fairy Liquid, and the job was oxo. Insert any used and oiled tissues or kitchen paper in the bottom of the rubbish bin, so as not to raise suspicions. Pour all used oil into a metal pot that had preferably spent the afternoon in the freezer chilling its handles off, and then put oil and pot back into freezer to speed up the cooling process. Once properly chilled, pour oil back into bottles. (In the past, before I decided to chill the oil, I often poured the hot oil – which had not reached a decent level of coolness – back into the plastic bottle, only for the cheap, lousy bottle to melt, not in such a way as to leak or become unstable, but certainly enough for any decent chip detective to notice that what was once a strong phallic-shaped, if slightly stodgy, yellowy olive-coloured container was now a rendition of Humpty Dumpty mimicking the Leaning Tower of Pisa.) Then clean the chip pan, removing as much of the smelly oil that often hides in the nooks and crannies under the rim as possible, and put it back in the press. This only leaves the biggest nuisance of all, and the number-one crime-scene no-no – the residual aroma of chips – a book of evidence in itself, which can stay in an average house in Dublin for two bloody days if you don't take the right precautions.

So how do you fumigate a house that smells like the inside of a chip shop? Well, there are a number of fail-safe measures that experience has taught me definitely work. Top of the list? Shoe polish. The number-one smell remover this side of the Pecos. Simply clean and shine two or three pairs of shoes, and by the time you've finished, your humble abode will smell like the inside of a polish shop, and no amount of chip detectives and hot-oil sleuths will be any the wiser. Back in those days, we went through polish as quickly as we went through oil, with my mother regularly complaining that I was using too much shoe polish (which I thought was odd, because she never saw me shining shoes, or anything else, for that matter). In more recent times, I've discovered that making coffee is just as good, with the striking of matches (although you need a lot of them) a distant third. Very importantly, the whole process, from preparation through eating to clean-up, needs to be done with all doors and windows fully open.

This blinding obsession with the chips is probably the intro-ductory module to my compulsive personality, which hides occa-sionally behind a closed door somewhere in the underbelly of all my worldly problems. And, to be fair to my parents, who weren't slow on the uptake when I needed a doctor during my childhood, in those days they hadn't the luxury of a medical profession to consult with about children with chip peculiarities. Although, come to think of it, if medical science has caught up with my predicament, they probably would have been embarrassed to bring me to a potato shrink, saying: 'I tell you straight, doc, Junior's got a problem with the chips.'

Anyway, in those days, the problem with the chips was, while a little alarming, just another headache in the raising of children. Like most parents who hadn't yet got stuck into the child-psy-chology fad, obsessive-disorder literature and the 1-2-3 of Freud, anything unusual in a child, which couldn't be explained, good or bad, was a sign of difference, and something more to be celebrat-ed than brushed under the carpet. So there I was, the little fella who loved chips, struggling to carry the stigma of a big gaping hole in my psyche where a 'chip fantasist' had apparently moved in. 'Ah, sure, isn't he lovely? Did you know he loves chips?'

Once, when I was a fourteen, my mother got me a four-stone bag of potatoes as part of my provisions when she and the rest of the family went off on a family holiday. I, luckily, was considered to be too old and, by that stage, too awkward, to be easily accommodated on the O'Doherty annual family jolly. Looking back, it seems like I ate chips for breakfast, dinner, tea and supper and spent all day watching the West Indies – Viv Richards, Larry Gomes and Desmond Haynes – batter the English around Edgbaston, Trent Bridge and Lords. It was a life of emerging decadence and my awakening as a genuine couch potato. Not surprisingly, from an educational perspective, by this stage of my development, while I didn't know one end of a hammer from the next, I could play a potato peeler backwards. Incidentically, my mother also hid the potato peeler more often than she hid the rest of the chip-making essentials – something that never really inconvenienced me, particularly when a knife would as easily do the trick.

Speaking of holidays – and don't worry, I'll get back to Bordeaux in a moment – such has been my chip obsession that I once brought the family's grizzled chip pan on a teenage holiday, when the lads decided to go camping off Carne beach in County Wexford. The chip pan raised a few eyebrows, especially among the Guards, who stopped us at a checkpoint looking for a kidnap-gang and decided to search the boot. I can still see the Guard's face looking at us all standing at the side of the road, his hand shaking the chip pan up and down at the five of us, as if it was a magic wand that had just turned into a murder weapon and he was the brightest lamp in the constabulary. Says he in his best country detective's voice, 'What's this for?' 'Making chips,' says I, knowing that this wasn't what he wanted to hear. 'Don't be funny with me, sonny,' says he. 'I know it's for making chips. But what's it really for?' While my friends all looked at me as if I was the criminal in a police line-up with the whereabouts of Lord Lucan in my jocks, my friend's father, who was driving the car and us to the sunny south-east, intervened, taking the Guard to one side, explaining that I had a chip obsession and that I never left home without the chip pan, and that it might just be a good idea to turn a blind eye to any criminal activity if indeed any had taken place.

At which point the Guard let us go with the standard police greeting, 'I'll let you go this time', his face contorted following my gaze as the car sped off towards Inch. To this day, I've always regretted not getting that Guard's name, for I'm sure that, with his obvious qualities, he made Super if not Commissioner in the 1980s or 1990s.

Once we got to Carne, the much-maligned chip pan, when not doing its intended business – filling us campers up with home-made chips – moonlighted on the sun-kissed sand dunes as a wine cooler. Sadly, that famous old chip pan, golden yellow at the sides and coated in a lather of old oil, is buried somewhere on Carne beach. Every time I hear Leonard Cohen's 'Famous Blue Raincoat', which was 'torn at the shoulder', for some unclear reason I think of that bloody chip pan. Some day I'm going to grab hold of a decent metal detector and go looking on the south-east coastline for that sentimental old chip pan, which means as much to me as anything else in my miserable life. It's the sort of adventure that should cue a film sequel, bringing the world's most famous mutt out of retirement once more for *Lassie Finds the Chip Pan*.

Having said all that, I'm not the only one in the Western World with a chip obsession. If you had a mind to follow heroes, which I don't, back in the 1970s you could easily have found your favourite footballer, wrestler or pot-bellied detective curb-crawling in areas where chippers hung out. So much so that it was common knowledge that role models in those days were more likely to eat nearly as many chips as I did, which has you wondering if eating chips was a cultural phenomenon in itself. Surely some sociology student looking for an idea for a thesis could easily follow this up. Everybody from footballers to rock stars ate chips as their drug of choice, long before LSD, heroin and cocaine became fashionable. Hands up who remembers the football magazine *Shoot*'s regular feature which each week asked a famous footballer – while also sussing out 'What's your favourite player, team and rock chick?' – 'What's your favourite food?' And I bet you know what the answer was too. Yes, chips. I'm sure the reporter who was assigned to the interview every week didn't even bother to ask the question but just filled in the answer. Who in their right mind wasn't eating chips? It was undoubtedly a cultural phenomenon. Although, credit where credit is due, there was talk at one time or other that Malcolm Allison – he of the lucky Fedora hat, large cigars and sheepskin coat – once tried to introduce pasta to the English footballer's diet, along with champagne and a packet of Havana cigars.

Strangely enough – and I don't want to seem as though I spend my time thinking up ideas for dissertations – a comparison between what *Shoot*'s footballers saw as their favourite food in the 1970s and footballers' dietary restrictions in the 1980s chronicles the metamorphosis of the fatty, chip-loving, typically bulky English centre-forward, like Malcolm McDonald or Bob Latchford, into the sniper pint-size penne-pasta strikers, like Gary Lineker and Peter Beardsley. From an Irish perspective, although I was never an Arsenal supporter, I was well aware that Liam Brady's nickname was 'Chippy Brady' when he arrived in London in the early 1970s, not so much because the brilliant number seven could chip a ball from any distance onto a sixpence but because he had an obsession with the old spuds in oil. And, interestingly, while German centre-forward Horst Hrubesch, a real horse of a man, whose early and late goals decided the 1980 European Championships in Italy, was known by the rather clumsy nickname 'Das Kopfball-Ungeheuer' (the Header Beast), his predecessor in the German national team, Gerd Müller, who was better known as 'Bomber der Nation' (the Nation's Bomber), was also known as 'Kleines Dickes Müller' (Short, Fat Müller), a pseudonym we can be assured didn't come from him munching the fatty bits out of a bag of chips.

In fact, on the subject of Germans and their chips, one night on a Spanish campsite many moons ago, my wife and I, as we sipped our way through a bottle of Ribera del Duero, were approached by three Germans – two guys and a girl – from an adjoining wooden bungalow. For three days, we'd observed and waved at the youngish threesome across from us, trying to figure out if the girl was with the little fat bald guy, whose head and face she meticulously and lovingly shaved early each morning and subsequently anointed and massaged with various creams, or the thinner vampire-ish moodier bloke, whom she kissed and cuddled up against during the late afternoon and early evening. It was classic François Truffaut *Jules et Jim* on the stage of a wooden chalet, with the two men living the bohemian free-loving existence, swapping the love of their beloved for their own personal friendship. Or maybe she was the puppet-master, toying with her two friends, coquettishly playing one off against the other, pillaging from these two different personalities the characteristics that made up her perfect man. Whatever the story, it was clear to my mind at least that she was the type of Catherine or Jeanne Moreau, who one day could easily entice one of her lovers to drive the pair of them over a bridge to their deaths.

So, sitting as we were on our veranda deciphering and distinguishing the mulberry-blackberry aromas from the richer fruits of the forest that were fast evacuating our glasses, we gasped as our neighbours, having approached in the darkness, wondered if they could ask us a delicate personal question. Imagining that the threesome was about to announce that they would like to become five, we gulped fast on our wine, glanced at each other in apprehension and told them to 'ask away'. 'Is it true,' says the modern-day Jules, 'that you Irish put vinegar on your chips?' Our reply had the three twenty-somethings rolling around on our veranda, while we poured another glass of wine, relaxed in the knowledge that our suspicions about their intentions were wide of the mark.

Not that footballers and Germans were the only people interested in chips. The cultural phenomenon also inspired comic heroes like *Tough of the Track*'s Alf Tupper, the working-class runner who made his name in the *Rover* before transferring to the *Victor*. It is from his time in the *Victor* that I remember Alf, taking on the clean-living, pompous AAAs college boys, with their fancy runners, kit and *Chariots of Fire* haircuts, and overcoming all sorts of ailments and bias in his puny tough-as-Norman-Hunter's-boots frame to grind out an underdog's victory in the illustrious meets around Europe. No matter whether he won or lost, Alf would always finish a race to the death with a bag of fish and chips served in yesterday's newspaper in some dilapidated chip shop in Blighty. Was there ever a more famous welder?

But that's all beside the substantive point, which is that, after about an hour and a half of frogmarching the wife around a wet Bordeaux, we found a suitable restaurant – one that served chips – Le Mably, a real old-fashioned French brasserie, painted green, with lace curtains in the windows and small lamps outside. Inside was like your aunt's sitting room, a lot smaller than it looked, the mirrors on the walls adding depth, which the burgundy ceiling removed. No sooner were we seated than a large American with a big pair of tinted 1970s sunglasses and a bigger wig – he looked like the Big O's older, obese brother – could be overheard complaining that there was too much duck on the menu. I wondered for a moment was he referring to the starter or the main courses, or perhaps the waiter had spilt his dinner over the menu. Duck, I thought to myself, lovely jubbly, my food horns bursting the balloons in my imagination as I dreamed up in an instant a hundred ways to have duck, served with or without chips. It was a good time to be a fat person with a big bulging, empty stomach. Hunger had dug a pit the size of Kenya in my stomach, and the muscles in my abdomen were already clearing a hotel of rooms for the arriving food. Usually, in these circumstances, I reach across the table and tell my wife that I love her and that 'This is the only time on the holiday I'm going to have chips and, I promise, when I say this I mean it'. Usually, she relents on my piggery for one night – provided it's the first night of the holiday – seeing in my eyes a contrite exterior that belies the devil within.

Knowing that I'm looking in the mirror at my conscience has its pluses and minuses. For the most part, I'm getting what I want in terms of food, my wife, like my conscience, giving in to my whims to keep the peace. Conversely, I'm lying to myself and storing up medical grief for the future. My wife knows it, my conscience knows it, and I know it. Unfortunately, only my wife really cares. For her, looking back at me across the table, unaware that she's my conscience, she probably sees a moment of contentment that won't get in the way of our food until, an hour later, overburdened with the dinner, I'm wondering to her, as much to as to myself, why I've overeaten again.

You might think that my wife shouldn't be telling a grown man what he can or can't eat, but you see, she's my conscience, my inner voice telling me what I should be hearing but am choosing to ignore. Like anyone crippled with a disease, I also need a crutch, someone to pick up the pieces, someone to draw the lines of normality in my everyday life. I'm obviously a retard in these circumstances, unable to decipher a path between any two lines of civility. Thus, in our house, my wife is in charge of laundry and morale. Laundry is a cute term for everything that involves cleaning, something my conscience repeatedly tells me I don't do well enough. I'd like to think that if I was ever forced to undergo severe psychometric testing to prove my ability at house-cleaning, I'd fail miserably, with scientific reams of paperwork to confirm it.

That's not to say that I'm dirty – far from it. In fact, I'm cleaner than most. It's just that cleaning in the nooks and crannies and getting down to floor level isn't my strong point, certainly not at my weight. OK, so I can carry a vacuum cleaner up and down stairs, and I don't mind taking it for a walk. Yes, it is tiring, but hey, it's better than using a sweeping brush.

Anyway, the restaurant starts to fill up, and we read the menu, my wife eyeing up an adventurous salad and me looking discreetly for whatever comes with chips. The starter is easy: it has to be foie gras, or 'fat liver', in English – particularly appropriate since, as I've mentioned, I've been attending the liver clinic in Dublin for the last four years, suffering from, you've guessed it – fatty liver.

However, sitting there in the Bordeaux restaurant with my conscience/wife, the starter arrives, and I've forgotten all about my next appointment with the liver doc. The food looks gorgeous, and I'm already digging into the bread and toast before I remember to ask the waiter for a glass of Sauternes, a lovely sweet accompaniment to the slender slice of duck liver. Two glasses of champagne later, and my wife is on the Bordeaux – a nice deep-garnet Château Coquillas, named for the exorbitant number of shells found in the soil on the parcel of land where the vines are grown, and the second wine of Château de France – gets an extra quarter-glass in compensation, for my Sauternes, to accompany her large goat's-cheese salad, which acts as both her starter and main course. By the time I've devoured the foie gras and am already on to my second basket of bread, the wife is begging me to go easy, and certainly not to order a third one. My chateaubriand arrives *à la bordelaise*, with a miserly portion of chips, the sauce running wild, reminding me that I'll need at least three more slices of bread to mop up the leftovers at the end of the meal, a view I immediately share with the wife, in case there's any misunderstanding when the time comes to order it. She reluctantly agrees, this once adding a disclaimer: 'Don't think you're going to eat yourself through Bordeaux – not with me, anyway.' By the end of the meal, and €90 later, I'm already finding it difficult to get out of the chair and put on my coat without catching my fat, ugly face in the multitude of mirrors which resembles the hall-of-mirrors finale in *Enter the Dragon*.

Outside, it has stopped raining, and it's 10.30 PM. We make our way down to the carnival which is down the street from our hotel. It's a really big carnival and takes up the whole of the Esplanade des Quinconces – a huge plot of land in the centre of Bordeaux that runs down to the River Garonne. Conscious that the brief weekend away is also an opportunity to restart an exercise spree, we decide to walk around the esplanade a few times, to shift a bit of the podge – *my* podge – before bedtime, wisely passing up on the candy floss that seems to be being sold on every second stall. The smell of overcooked burgers and fries is everywhere, and almost give me a second hunger. I'm stopped by the lingering face in the mirror which looked back at me as I left the restaurant, a sad, bloated countenance, unhappy with the food packed solid in the storeys below. As we make our way three-quarters of the way around the carnival, the amusements slowly switch off, closing down the first night of our holiday in Bordeaux.

The following morning, we wake about seven to a full hour of rapid fire muffled chute-ing coming in the window. Chute-ing? Yes, chute-ing. Chute, chute, chute, chute, bang. Chute, chute, chute, chute, bang. I jump out of bed and leg it over to the window, where, to the right of the hotel and six doors down, a team of labourers from eight or nine storeys up – obviously I can't be totally accurate, because I'm hanging out of the window – are firing rubble, stone and slate out of a window rhythmically, as if René the Builder is standing behind them with a metronome, down one of those builders' loop-the-loop matchbox-style roller-coasters – which normally accessorise activity swimming pools – into a massive skip below. Retching, retching, vomiting – an unwanted air-conditioning unit misses out on a trip to the recyclers and explodes in a mess of stone below me to the right. It's quickly followed by an old fireplace and a silver-haired ducting unit, half a mile long. Dust recreates 9/11 while the French below, conveniently, enter and leave the smog at breakfast time. Retch, retch, vomit – the noise follows me all the way back to bed, where the wife has sequestrated the spare pillow to cover her ears. 'Jaysus,' I say to the wife, 'do they not know we're on fucking holiday?'

At 9 am, a skip arrives to replace the first skip, which is now overflowing. Bang, bang, boof, bang, boof, bang, the skip is taken away by an over-brake-conscious driver, and it's nearly time to get our breakfast, considering that we're on French time and lunch is potentially only 180 minutes away. By the time I'm washed, showered and dressed, and waiting for my wife to hurry up so we can get down to the *petit déjeuner* before all the croissants are gone, the pounding of the early morning has been replaced by the meandering, winding drift of a cellist practising and re-practising Dvořák, one or two floors below, serenading the distressed hotel congregation. Jesus, I say to myself, if it's not an earthquake, it's a fucking anaesthetic. And how do I know it's Dvořák? Well, I'll get to that in a minute.

Scale up, scale down, the music winds its way around the inner staircase, a Pied Piper calling me to breakfast. 'Hurry up, love, I'm starving.' I give the wife a reminder that breakfast is served until 10 AM and that, at nearly 9.50 AM, we're bound to run into trouble downstairs. 'Come on, hurry up! There'll be nothing left.' Eventually she's ready to go, and we descend into the foyer, the rumble in my stomach energised by the cellist. In the dining room, breakfast seems to be finished, as French, English and Oriental dudes hover over what looks like the remains of the croissants and coffee, passing sheets of music back and forth. On the ground beside them lie music cases of various sizes. Amidst the babble of voices, Dvořák, Mendelssohn and Grieg jump across the table to me as I send the wife off to find out about our breakfast. The musicians – I assume they're all musicians, since they're in a hotel with its own personal elevator-music, where the male cellist is still playing Dvořák, and around the corner is The Grand Theatre – speak a little in French, a little in English, a little more in French. I earwig snippets. Apart from an Oriental in the corner drinking his coffee over a breadbasket – and I can't emphasise the breadbasket enough at this juncture, the wheels on my hunger are close to falling off – the five musicians, and my wife, who has gone missing, the room is deserted.

The wife comes back with a tray bearing two glasses of orange juice, four miserable-looking croissants, enough bread to feed four flies for a day and two mugs of coffee. 'Is that it?' I ask, realising that there's not even enough food for me. 'It's all that's left,' she says, 'and it's probably enough. And, sure, it's only a few hours to your lunch.' She says 'your lunch' as if I'm the only one getting fed today. It's micro-speak for fat people. Looking to the future, it's only a matter of time before fat people are refused drink in pubs and lose the right to hold wedding receptions in hotels.

Understanding, however, that this is no time for a debate, I tuck in. I've no sooner swallowed the orange juice than two of the croissants – one of which has just enough chocolate in its *pain au chocolat* to die for – have gone for a hop, and I'm already eating my share of the rolls. By the time I've finished my coffee, the wife has had only one roll and one croissant, and has very kindly given me the last croissant. It's not enough. Breakfast is the main meal of the day, they say, and you've never heard a truer word, particularly when looking into the oblivion of an empty plate. The cellist appears to be reaching a musical hiatus and is definitely getting a little louder – and getting on my nerves, adding another layer to my hunger. I'm not a violent man, but I want to go upstairs and throttle him, letting him know in the strongest possible terms what happens when at least one of the other guests hasn't had a proper breakfast.

When the Oriental leaves his table, the wife and I are the only ones left in the room. I spy that he has left a full basket of bread rolls, which from a distance doesn't look to have been touched, and has my name on it. I convince my wife to go over and get the bread, which she does after a slight 'No, you go and get them', followed by my 'Don't be stupid, you're closer, and anyway I'm stuck in here on the inside and I'll probably make too much noise getting over there fast enough.' The bread is wonderful, plentiful and succulent. It's not what you'd call a full Irish, but it's tasty and filling. I dig in with gusto.

Unfortunately, the Oriental hasn't gone, and returns to the table a minute of two later with another cup of coffee. He stares across a foodless table for the basket of rolls he knows was there a few minutes ago. His basket now empty, I sit back and try to ignore a potential international incident as the wife tries to hide her face in shame, and suggests we offer an explanation. 'What are you going to say?' I ask. 'My husband's an absolute pig and he encouraged me to go over and nick your breakfast. And I'm sorry, I don't know the French for "absolute pig". Not on my watch,' I say, hurriedly grabbing the wife before she can make an apology, reminding her that we booked a private tour of Bordeaux with the tourist office for 10.30 AM and we're already late.

Outside the Office de Tourisme, we meet our tour guide for the trip around Bordeaux. Véronique is well kitted out in walking shoes, lightish clothing and coat, cleverly dressed for every eventuality. I, on the other hand, am wearing a heavy, albeit new, pair of trousers, which are already beginning to hot up, causing my jockeys to stick to my undercarriage in the moderate heat, and a shirt and jacket that are probably more suited to a day that is a couple of degrees colder. A tram ride later, my wife and I – the only two on the tour – are following our pathfinder around the back streets of old Bordeaux, stopping to view reference points, representative houses and churches, and ongoing redevelopment and various refurbishments, taking us out onto the Quai des Chartrons on the west bank of the Garonne, where for centuries the Bordeaux wine trade was cellared. It's a decent warm morning and fairly quiet, save for the obvious fact that the municipal powers are upgrading the road and path network along the quay, and for a couple of miles it's virtually all a building site.

This wouldn't be too bad if Véronique, whose English is word-perfect and whose tour is very informative, wasn't on a mission to show us as much of her city as was humanly possible within the allotted time or had a walking speed for the obese as well as one for Olympic sprinters. I'm convinced that we're on world-record time and that some official in a blue blazer is going to tip me on the shoulder to tell me I'm walking the fifty-kilometre discipline illegally and that I'm out of the race. No such luck, as the march continues, the jockeys filling up on the spare sweat that's evacuating the glands that cushion my wobbly bits. Trying to walk in such a way as would allow me not to have to feel the wetness in my groin area attracts Véronique's attention. She asks me if I'm enjoying the walk, aware that I'm carrying my legs like a ventriloquist's dummy. 'Oh, yes,' I reply – which I am – declining to tell her that my mind has momentarily jumped from the history lesson to a recollection of all the places where I suffered with sweat, most notably the time I was in hospital for a knee operation. Yes, that was the time when my mother bought me a pair of burgundy pyjamas, reminding me that if I was going into hospital overnight, I'd need something to wear. Like most blokes my age, I go commando when I go to bed, unable to have even a smidgen of clothing near my body when I jump under the covers. Not that I haven't had the odd skid-mark or two to explain to the wife over the years, although I've had moderate success in cleaning them with toothpaste. If you don't believe me, try it.

Anyway, going in for the knee operation, I was putting on pyjamas for the first time in more than fifteen years and, while conscious that I had to obey hospital rules, I wasn't entirely happy about the idea. However, I did what I had to do and, after the knee job, was moved to a room to recuperate overnight. Morphine-induced, I had one of the best nights of my life, waking up in the middle of the night to be told by a nurse that I could have some toast and butter if I felt up to it. 'Toast? Yes, thank you,' I said, 'but no butter', not having taken butter on anything since I was a child. The unbuttered toast duly arrived, a feast fit for a king. Months later, when I got the bill from the hospital, I was invoiced for everything from the bed to the four tablets of morphine and various other pills. Such was the preciseness of the bill, I was also charged for one slice of toast, and two pence for butter. The trouble I had convincing the hospital that a mistake had been made on the invoice and that, no, I shouldn't have been charged for the spread. In the end, they send me a credit note for the two pence, and I duly paid up.

But that's a deviation from the story. There I was having a good night's sleep after the knee job and the toast when I woke up around eight the following morning in a lather of sweat and bursting for a jimmy riddle. Out of the bed I jumped, and hopped across the room to the ensuite, with a book I had by the bed, and a spare pair of jockeys. Soaking everywhere, I stripped off and threw everything into the bath, had a quick wash, and got down to business. About fifteen minutes later, having made myself comfortable on the pot, I heard screaming from the bedroom. Pulling up my clean trunks, I hopped back into the room to find a nurse looking at my bed with her hands up to her face, screaming hysterically while two more nurses rushed into the room, wondering what in the name of jaysus was going on in Room 12. 'What's wrong?' I asked, hoping that the other two nurses didn't think I had tried something on with their colleague. Turning around, the nurse pointed at me like you'd point at Lazarus coming out of the tomb. 'You're not dead,' she says. 'Thank God, you're alive. Look at the bed!' says she, 'it's after frightening the life out of me.' This I and the two other nurses had to see. Looking into the bed, the outline of Leonardo da Vinci's Vitruvian Man had been ironed into the bed in a deep red burgundy, although from where I was standing – beginning to suffer cold turkey from my nascent dependency on morphine – I wasn't sure if my wobbly bits were missing. 'What happened to the bed?' they said collectively, rushing towards me to check me out for cuts. 'Are you bleeding?' Hopping on one leg, and self-conscious that I was wearing only a pair of skimpy jocks, I had a hard job explaining to the nurses that I had been sweating all night and my burgundy pyjamas had run. 'Jesus,' says one of nurses, 'you must sweat like a right pig.'

Yes, I said to myself, standing in a wet pair of jockeys under a heavy pair of trousers on the Quai des Chartrons, *you're right: I definitely sweat like a pig.* But before I had time to contemplate a moment of pity, we were off again on another 1,500-metre dash up past Quinconces, Place de la Bourse and Place du Palais, Véronique expatiating on the architecture, period houses and various snippets of fascinating history. Three hours later, knackered and sweating like the bejaysus, we said goodbye and returned to our hotel for a much-needed shower, declining to tell Véronique that she was missing her vocation as a personal trainer. Forget fat clubs, Weightwatchers, the Southeast Beach Diet, The Diet Channel and Overeaters Anonymous. If you're seriously interested in losing weight, take a mid-week break in Bordeaux and book a tour around the city. You're bound to lose the guts of ten pounds.

We went out for lunch to the Café Gourmand (a good recommendation if you're in Bordeaux) on rue Buffon, where I had arranged to meet a contact for lunch. Starving from the walk of walks, I was forced to hold back, reluctantly not wanting to make a pig of myself in front of a stranger. I've always found it much more difficult to really get stuck in when I meet someone new over a meal for the first time, and even at subsequent meetings, at least until I get to know them. So, while the food was superb, I can't say I had what I really wanted – certainly not in the quantities that a three-hour walk at speed had inspired. We had already signed up for a wine tasting at one of Bordeaux's best cheese restaurants, where I was hoping that, while I wasn't a great lover of cheese, I could at least have a go at the nibbles that went with it. Restaurant Baud et Millet on rue Huguerie is a tight little eatery with plenty of old-world charm and two well-stocked cellars of wine and cheese. The wine lesson over, our group of about sixteen people was invited – for the price of the admission – into the cool cheese cellar in the basement to take as much cheese as we could humanly eat before it was time to go. For cheese-lovers, and my wife is one of them, this is a Mecca on the tour of the region. While the rest of the party were scampering in and out of the glass-covered cave like Ali Baba and the Forty Thieves, taking full advantage of the restaurant's generosity, I sat back for a moment and watched the behaviour that I'm normally famous for, not afraid for once to look in the mirror – metaphorically speaking, you understand.

What you might call a Bordeaux takeaway – baguette, ham and tomato, and a bottle of wine from La Vinothèque de Bordeaux – later, after sitting in my underpants looking out over the rooftops across the street as the sun slipped from the sky, we dressed in our glad rags and went out for an evening at the Grand Theatre to hear the Orchestre National Bordeaux Aquitaine perform Dvorák's *Concerto pour violoncelle en si mineur* and an overture by Mendelssohn. By the time the conductor, Yutaka Sado, had ripped into his night's entertainment, I realised that what I had been hearing in the hotel all morning was now somewhere on stage. I'm already planning what I'm going to have for my supper when Sado turns to bow to the audience and milk the applause, and I recognise him immediately. 'Jesus,' I say to the wife, without realising how loud I am, 'that's the Oriental whose breakfast we took this morning.' A raised *Sssh!* reacts angrily to my outburst, and we both slink sheepishly out of the concert hall in embarrassment.

For the next two days we ate, dined and drank our way around the city, visiting vineyards Sauternes and Graves, among other districts, and lapping up the warm spring weather. Thoughts of exercise had long since been exorcised, and by the time we arrived back in Dublin airport, the only serious workout I'd had in Bordeaux, apart from the walk of a lifetime, was the movement involved in taking the luggage on and off the trolley.

MAY

GYM'LL FIX IT?

By May, I feel like I'm already another third of the way into a further year of desperation, and I'm still the big fat lad with the parachute trousers, double chin and humpty-dumpty wobble. I hand in my notice to F-Troop, and the society of perpetual losers. It just hasn't worked, and I can see clearly it isn't for me. I'm not taken in by all the hype, minor-league psychology and feel-good buddyism that works very successfully for a lot of people. I begin to think I need to get a little more sophisticated, spend a little more money on improving my circumstances, and considerably up the ante. It's a month to the summer holidays and I'm nowhere near any level of even moderate fitness, and my shape continues to be the fat side of square. I decide to take drastic action and join a local gym. The Conscience joins too: a family pack, you could call it, his and hers. We go shopping. T-shirts, shorts, white socks and runners later, we're walking side by side, like joined-at-the-hip Americans on a conveyer-belt, watching Sky Sports, various news channels and music stations on the wall in the distance, the sound cut, while a local radio signal beams in, in stereo, giving voice to a pair of Muppets you wouldn't persecute prisoners with in Guantánamo Bay, for fear of being accused of human-rights abuses.

It's monotonous, boring drudgery. Pound, pound, pound. Walking going nowhere into a television screen is about as interesting as imaginary dinners, and you just want to jump off and go find the bastard who invented this preposterous form of treadmilling and chain him to a radiator in Beirut or Terry Waite's old bicycle outside Canterbury Cathedral. Boring, boring, boring.

Endlessly bloody boring. Am I the only one complaining? Apparently yes. Everybody else in the gym appears to be in a hurry to go somewhere fast, sweat spilling from their glands like mobile water hydrants fitted around their bodies. There's an underground collegiality that I don't feel a part of. To the front, the grave-dodgers are lined up in their Persil-white T-shirts pedalling bikes that are going nowhere slowly, while for every tier of exercise bike, treadmill and leg-ski you go back, you may as well have asked the membership to line up in descending order according to the decade of their birth. It's either that or the younger members seem to have better eyesight to watch the television screens. It's exercise-trials by media, and you just know that in five years' time, anyone considering membership will ask legitimately of a gym manager, before joining, if the warm-up bikes have broadband capability or if there are personal plasma screens on the treadmill desktops.

Regardless, I try a little harder, getting myself into the mood, inspired by all the athletes around me. I switch on the treadmill's computer and key in my weight (I guess 181 kgs – I'm sure it doesn't matter), age and speed (I try five kilometres an hour – how fast can 5k an hour be?). The treadmill takes on a mind of its own. It's apparently going for a run, and taking me with it, the black lino below me forcing my legs to move like fuck. I nearly fall, and grab hold of the rails for dear life, as the computer on my dashboard tells me it's an offence to hold the rails. *No way*, I say back, *I'm fucked if I'm taking any chances on a machine with a plug.* Forty-one minutes later, I'm rather chuffed with myself. OK, so my arms are nearly as sore as my legs, but I've gone a little over 5 miles, deprived myself of a bucket-load of sweat and, according to the know-all computer, lost 800 calories, which, a gym instructor in passing tells me as I finish, 'amounts to about eight and a half cans of Coke'. It hardly seems worth it, and this feeling is compounded when the wife, next door, puts in her oar by telling me that I had entered the wrong weight, that I'm not 181 kilograms; closer maybe to 110 kgs. Suddenly, I realise why I'd never wanted to be a politician: the dreaded recount. Instead of eight and a half cans of Coke, it's nearer to five – what you might call a reduced majority. So, five cans of Coke later, I'm thinking that the gym is totally ridiculous and that forty minutes of jogging is only a baby rung on the ladder up Walton's Fat Mountain. That night, reading Nicholas Stargardt's *Witnesses of War: Children's Lives Under the Nazis*, I come across a worrying stat that says that the average daily ration to barely stay alive in a concentration camp in 1943 was 800 calories a day. Jesus, I say to myself, and I'm complaining that I didn't quite lose that amount – enough to keep a person alive sixty-odd years ago.

Getting off the treadmill, I nearly lose my balance: I'm disorientated and goggle-eyed from watching the coterie of mute screens. I steady myself and walk around the room. I'm in serious trouble. I want to give up, stop off at the chipper on the way home and stack up on at least two snack boxes. For some reason, I don't. I grab my bottle of water, which is nearly empty, and go into what they call the quiet room for some cool-down time and a few stomach and back exercises. There are four other people there, and all are considerably thinner than me. I wonder do they live there. When we joined – the Conscience and I – we told the instructor we wanted to lose weight, obviously, but also to loosen out around the midriff. Only a day after getting private tuition, I've forgotten everything I've learned. The instructor – a young, attentive college girl, studying medicine or home economics, when she's not paying for her tuition in the gym – asked all the right questions of me, including, to the wife's annoyance, 'Have you worked out before? It looks like it.' My wife smiled back an exaggerated grin and mimicked the words for the rest of the day. '"Have you worked out before?" she asks. Is she blind? You're over seventeen stone, with two chins and an arse that a Morris Minor could hide in, and she asks, "Have you worked out before?" Is she out of her mind? And, before you start, don't flatter yourself. She's only doing her job. I bet she says that to all the fellas. And what did you say? "Oh, yes", Mr Bloody Important, "of course I once worked out extensively in my youth." "Extensively in my youth" – what does that mean? You'd want to cop yourself on.'

I try to compose myself. I lie down on my back on a mat and bend my legs at the knees and put my hands on my head. I remember that I'm supposed to raise my head off the floor and at the same time feel the pressure around my stomach. It doesn't come easy, and only for another bloke coming into the room and disturbing the quietness, I'm close to nodding off, you understand. Physically knackered.

Anyway, I start, aiming to do about ten stomach crunches at a go. No sooner have I got to two than I'm starting to fart. Not little silent ones that I'm sure keep the postulants awake at night in convents but rocket-launchers that you could fire at the Taliban. Three, four – SPLUT. Five – SPLUT, SPLUT. Six, seven – SPLUT, SPLUT, SPLUT. I stop, mortified with embarrassment. I'm the only one in the mirrored room lying on the ground, and the only one making any noise. And it's involuntary; I've no control over my movements. While no one in the room objects, I feel I should say something, anything. I even prepare a little speech: *I'm terribly sorry for all that. Totally out of character. Sort of just happened. Hope I didn't cause anyone too much discomfort. And I can promise you solemnly it will never happen again.*

But I don't say it. I lie absolutely still and hope that everyone is deaf or even hard of hearing and that they imagine they are making noise and feel uncomfortable thinking about it. And off I go again, praying that the farting will stop. Eight. Luckily, nothing. Nine – SPLUT, SPLUT. *Oh no*, I say to myself. Ten – SPLUT, SPLUT, SPLUT, SPLUT, SPLUT, SPLUT. It's probably the worst noise you can hear, never mind smell, when you're working out. Although, now that I think of it, the sound of keys jangling when I'm exercising really annoys me as well. Anyway, I've had enough and try desperately to get up off the floor as quickly as possible and leave. It's not easy. I'm so big, I have trouble getting up in one movement, and have to roll to one side and then pop up, as you would imagine a baby seal might do if he fell coming home from the shops with his mother's messages.

Downstairs in the men's changing room, I notice that many of the fat blokes are wearing miserably old-looking towels in various shades of yellow which don't quite fit the rumps that men of such stature deserve. A number of them have stretch-marks high on their waists from trying to pull their towels tight, as you would a belt, giving the impression that they've experienced childbirth and are likely to experience it again in the future. They're also complaining of stomach pains, liver abnormalities and hypertension, when all they need is to change their towels. I, on the other hand, am hidden in the largest towel possible, with enough width for even Yogi Bear to store a year's supply of honey, jam and EPO for the Tour de France, and not raise a hair of suspicion among commissars, director sportifs or fickle journos.

Anyway, what's with the fetish for yellow towels? You seriously wonder if any of these blokes have ever seen *Ben Hur*, with probably the most famous male towel scene in history – up until *Top Gun*, that is. I'm sure everybody remembers that when Sheik Ilderim (played so impressively by Hugh Griffith) makes an appearance in the Roman baths to wind up Messala (Stephen Boyd) and the rest of the masters of the universe with the 'Roman better than a Jew' speech, all the Romans are dressed in white mass-produced towels, probably manufactured in some sweatshop toga factory in Sicily. Do people not learn? How many of the Romans had yellow towels? Or, in *Top Gun*, did Ice, Viper, Goose or Yester deface flight school by wearing yellow towels? *The hard-deck on this hop will be conducted in yellow towels.* No, they didn't. It leaves you wondering if the Irish male has been traumatised from playing Lego and having to watch *The Multi-coloured Swap-shop*. Or, if you're being desperately unkind, you could say that yellow towel syndrome (YTS) is probably caused by the reaction the men folk get from the wife, girlfriend, sister or mother when they tell them they're going training and does it matter which towel they take. I bet you most men in this situation are told: 'Take the yellow towel in the back of the hot press. Yes, the one Aunty what's-her-name gave us for Christmas in 1979.' How many people in Ireland got presents of yellow towels in 1979, presumably leftovers from the Pope's visit – the papal colours and all that? And how many were given a wedding present from the next-door neighbour, who, while not invited to the nuptials themselves, still felt obliged to buy a small wedding present – a set of yellow towels – that same year? Don't be surprised when the Mahon Tribunal, or the tribunal after that one, ends, and the one man ultimately responsible for all the corruption in this country is discovered to have made his money from flogging yellow towels in 1979, and since. Not that that is the only reason why men end up with yellow towels in Ireland. Walk into any linen department in Ireland, particularly during the sales, and the only men buying towels are parish priests.

Anyway, for a month, that was the routine. Up to the gym, ten minutes on the bike, forty minutes on the treadmill, and twenty minutes doing the stomach exercises. Shower, wash, shave and home. (Surprisingly, for the thirty days I did this, I was the only person I ever saw shaving. Now I've nothing against people shaving at home, but I felt it a bit odd that they never once shaved in the gym, particularly since they were washing themselves there at the time. I also must point out that I was only in the gym for one hour a day, and only in the changing rooms for ten minutes during the same time: it wouldn't stand up as a piece of research, if you know what I mean.)

Monday mornings are the worst mornings for pounding the treadmill. It's usually been a hectic weekend. A few drinks on Friday night, the same on Saturday, and just when I've squeezed in the last morsel of the last bit of grub on Sunday night, I get a goo for alcohol and before I know it I'm drooling into my drink, telling the world how great I am. That is until early the following morning in the gym when, spurting and farting, I'm bursting my arse running in tandem with the weight-management suffragettes. Until the fitness instructors appear with their polish and shimmies and start wiping the imaginary spots to the left and right on the treadmills' screen keyboard. Fart, fart, fart, I'm gasping for air and making the slow grind up the hill on the first kilometre and unable to steady myself long enough to drink from my still-full bottle of water; the shimmy brigade make matters worse by infecting the atmosphere with enough spray to close Sellafield. And not to be outdone, the 'new boy' appears with the vacuum cleaner, terrified that someone will tell his mammy that he was seen with a vacuum-cleaner hose around his neck taking the fat mechanical sausage for a walk. Spot-cleaning the carpet like any ordinary bloke forced to do women's work (the sheer indignity of it), he's soon under my feet, head down like a mountain biker on a roll and smelling the odours that are leaking from my direction. Looking up, he makes one of those 'you smelly bastard' gestures, pursing his lips. 'It wasn't . . . me', I inform him with an out-of-breath stutter. 'I think . . . it's . . . coming from the vacuum cleaner.' Switching it off, he stares down the barrel of the gun for inspiration: it's definitely his first time hoovering.

Tuesdays, Wednesdays, Thursdays, Fridays, Saturdays and Sundays. It becomes a bit of an obsession, and you can see the difference. Within thirty-odd days, while I can't really say that I've lost tons of weight – I haven't – I've definitely changed shape: I'm less square, more rectangular, and my chin and face muscles are toning up. And I certainly feel a lot more flexible, and even a little prouder of the old body. However, there's much more to it than that. The going-nowhere syndrome of treadmilling is still freaking me out, and I'm beginning to suffer slight headaches, bouts of dizziness, and pain attacks during my five-kilometre run. I'm convinced these are caused by the monotonous nature of what I'm doing, and glaring at the bloody television screens hanging in front of me.

I decide to take up swimming; the Conscience and I (another family pack) do the duck thing off to the twenty-five-foot pool, where we take proper lessons. Originally, my father taught me to swim when I was a nipper. Unfortunately, he used the Johnny Weissmuller method. This usually involved watching faint early-1930s to early-1940s black-and-white *Tarzan* movies, then wrestling for about an hour on our hard sitting-room floor. My dad told me that this was how you fought crocodiles, just in case in the wet swamplands of south-west Dublin an alligator or croc happened to make it inland from the canal, jaywalk its way across two main roads, dodge the nutters who were congregated outside the chipper, and then choose our house to pick a fight with me. This game usually finished if I beat my dad. If I didn't, there was a good chance we'd go swimming in the baths – what we now call the swimming pool.

In those days, the baths could be pretty busy, in particular the five o'clock Saturday session, which was manic. Off-peak was a much better option: with a bit of luck, we had the pool to ourselves. Here we practised the Johnny Weissmuller method, which meant swimming widths or lengths, or looking for hair-clips or pennies at the bottom the pool. You know, the usual: you find it, then I find it. As for the swimming, it probably looked a lot like splashing, or Johnny Weissmuller fighting the *crocodylus niloticus*. Within five minutes of my first lesson with my swimming instructor, I realised, in retrospect, that my father was probably a better crocodile wrestler than a swimming instructor. In fact, I'd hazard a guess that most Irish fathers are better crocodile wrestlers than swimming instructors.

So, there I was learning to swim properly with an instructor. Before I could swim the big lengths, she had me swimming four or five strokes – about twelve feet – from a distance out in to the bar. Initially it's all low-grade stuff, and I feel like I'm a toddler learning to paddle, in against the rail on my first day in the swimming pool. The instructor asks me which side of my nose do I breathe through? Which side do I breathe through? *Jesus*, I say to myself, *what language are you speaking?* 'I just take a deep breath and off I go.' 'No', she says, 'I mean when you're swimming lengths, do you prefer to take a breath on the right or on the left?' The right or the left? 'I just breathe straight ahead,' I say. This, I realise, is not the type of Pauly-speak she wants to hear, and after a more detailed examination of my swimming technique, I can see in her face – despite the fact that I'm wearing a pair of ill-fitting goggles that are wrapped around my face like a bandage where my prescription glasses should be – that she thinks I've as much swimming culture as a baby dolphin in a kebab shop.

The lesson appears easy. I'm to make my arms seem long, swing them athletically over my head as I swim with a bit of style and grace, but also slowly, and I must kick my feet. This makes no concession to the obvious fact that I'm over 17 stone, and chucking my arms over my head athletically and gracefully is as awkward a proposition as trying to put on or take off my jockeys. You see, flexibility is a big issue for a fat bloke. Yes, of course I want to do it, but the wobbly bits and the hardened fat deposits get in the way. It's like trying to get past a tractor on a country road. No matter how fast your engine is, if the big wheels are in the way, you're fucked. Aside from all that, I give it my best shot.

Start. One stroke, two strokes, three strokes, four strokes, reach bar. Return to starting point, and begin again. OK, so it's a little monotonous, but at least I feel like I'm going somewhere. After a while, I start to think: *if this is swimming, it's very easy.* After thirty minutes, I have it off by heart. Then the instructor revisits the breathing issue. We start off a little further out. 'Right,' she says. 'I want you to swim those four strokes, take a breath, and you can take it left or right' – I decide to breathe to my right, for whatever reason I don't know – 'and then swim another four strokes and take another breath.' It all seems really easy, until after four strokes I try taking a breath and it's impossible. My mouth, lungs, chin, head and brain all go swim-about and I can't get them thinking on the one wavelength. By the time I have completed the second four strokes, I'm out of breath and taking in water. Gulp, gulp, gulp, and I'm over to the side, spewing up my guts, which because I haven't eaten anything all morning – never eat before you swim, they told us – is made up of the noxious taste of chlorine and pool-water.

We do it again. I say *we*, but it's only me in the water; the instructor's walking along at the side of the pool. I'm also, as I've mentioned, wearing goggles for the first time since I started to wear glasses, and I find the whole adventure really frustrating. For one thing, I can't really see the instructor properly; she's sort of a roaring mirage above me in the rarefied artificial atmosphere of the swimming complex, which always sounds as if there's a major commotion going on around you. And I'm getting headaches – something I always get if I don't wear my glasses. Which is the least of my worries, the main one being that I just don't know how to breathe. It's seems madness, because I've been breathing since I was born. Even as a new-born baby I could do it – even before I knew I could do it, I could do it – but here, a 17-odd stone of uselessness, I've lost something that should come naturally to me.

We go again, another short length. And once again, my breathing doesn't happen. And again, and again, and again, by which time the instructor is shouting at me to breathe. 'Breathe! Breathe! Breathe!' she says, which from my perspective, with my face stuck in the water swimming forwards, sounds like 'Br– Br– Br–.

Br– Br– Br–.' I know she's shouting 'Breathe! Breathe! Breathe!' because every time I come up for air – although I'm supposedly not getting any, air I mean – I can hear her screaming hysterically 'Breathe! Breathe! Breathe!'

By the fifth lesson, though, I've learned to swim a little more gracefully, and I am no longer splashing. I've started to finish lengths, although I know I'm still not breathing right. And then it happens, as it was bound to happen. One, two, three, four – breathe. One, two, three, four – breathe. One, two, three, four – breathe. Achievements don't come any higher than this, and soon, after my ten minutes on the bike, forty minutes on the treadmill and twenty minutes doing the stomach exercises, I'm doing twenty minutes in the pool. It doesn't seem like an awful lot but I'm beginning to see a big difference in my dwindling face.

Aside from the other exercises, I take a teach-in in the gym itself, with all its bustling machines, weights and spinning classes. Despite one instructor saying that I looked like I worked out, I've been unlucky enough to be born with a frame that is easily disposed to that square shape that weights and over-exercise deform. And, yes, I did work out back in the days when the bow and arrow was a secret weapon, and got so far out of my natural shape that I swore I'd never use weights or weighing machines again. But this is different: I'm on a programme, so to speak. I try as many weights as I can – press-benches, lat machines, peck decks – and one particular monstrosity, a leverage chin-up and dip-assist machine that looks like Predator in his jocks. I use lowish weights because every time I try to get intense, another scourge of life – sciatica – pops up for a party, and ruins another day of exercise. Over the years, I've tried to clear up this problem at the physiotherapist's, where they've usually told me: 'Yes, you've a problem with your back, but we'll sort it out for you.' Two, three months later, I'm still attending their couch, being told: 'You do realise that you've got into this position from years of neglect, and don't think we'll be able to fix it overnight.' Well, actually I do, and I'm paying you far too much for that insight: do I look like I want to be attending you for the rest of my life? And so I leave, never to go back. Until the next time, and the next rendition of 'Does this hurt?', followed by the usual response of 'Aaagh! Yes of course it hurts, that's why I'm here', followed by 'Yes, you've a problem with your back, but we'll sort it out for you. Oh, and that will be fifty euro.'

Sciatica aside, I join a spinning class, one of those hour-long sessions where thirty or forty people go cycling to indoor music in what looks like someone's spare bedroom. The trouble is it's all artificial: you're going nowhere on what is a bony saddle, and if the guy next to you decides he'd prefer to wait all day for his spinning class before having a shower, you're in for a nauseating sixty minutes. Anyway, I try it for a while. In the mirrored room, the sight of my body on my bike is as revolting as seeing a pregnant pyramid, my chubby cheeks staring back at me, the pain of a hard slog written on my face. And I haven't even started cycling yet. The music starts. It's almost always a loud, raise-the-troops anthem from Freddie Mercury, Robbie Williams or U2, and it's expected that you'll cycle to the beat and the direction from the instructor. 'Up a turn,' the instructor bellows over the cacophony, a turn meaning a turn of a little knob down near the handlebars attached to the bike's wheels which determines the rate of difficulty it takes to turn the pedals, the music bouncing off the ceiling, my ears struggling to hear what she's saying. 'Up another turn,' I think she says. 'And another.'

By this stage you're supposed to be struggling – and I am – but because the term 'One more turn' has no objective meaning, there are still cyclists zooming along as if the incline is having no effect at all. Admittedly, they're losing buckets of sweat, and they look as if they're dying for some cause, but so am I, and yet my pedal power is draining from my legs. While I am reminiscent of Jan Ulrich going into oxygen debt during the Tour de France, there are guys around me pedalling like billy-o. As I struggle to turn the pedals, I think of Ulrich, a guy who arrived every year on the first day of the Tour looking like Billy Bunter, a fat bloke like myself who obviously loves his food and has had well-documented problems keeping his weight under control. Ulrich once claimed after a day's controversial racing that he had forgotten to eat. I'm not on the bike ten minutes and I'm thinking of my dinner, so whether or not you believe Ulrich's repeated cries that he never took drugs, he lost all credibility for me the day he protested that he forgot to eat. Not possible, Jan my boy, not possible.

By the time I'm finished, I'm wondering why someone doesn't fit an odometer and a calorie counter to the bikes during a spinning class, to see who has lost the most calories on what's supposed to be a spin. Getting off the bike, I've also realised that my hole feels as if four-foot monkeys have been head-butting me where the sun doesn't shine. Saddle-sore, I'm told, but later on in the year I'll realise that it's much more than exercise-related.

JUNE

HOLIDAYS IN FRANCE

For me, the annual holiday, and my desperation to overeat everything in sight, are just two interpretations of the same tune. And, so closely are they related, a psychologist would probably have trouble telling them apart, as if they were twin asparagus spears lying down in a bed of butter. It's almost as if the inner mechanisms of a countdown clock is always on the go, loudly flushing out my inner beast, like those women-folk who rattled their dustbin lids during the hunger strikes in the North. Trash, trash, trash, it goes. No matter, whether it's a dinner or a holiday, I always seem to be marching to the next great feast or trip, without really enjoying what's in front of me. Some people might put this down to boredom but I'm not the sort of person who gets bored easy. Far from it: I've more tricks than a circus of ponies, and enough hobbies, enjoyments and thrills in my life to fulfil ten people's dreams, and probably more if I was slimmer. So, once the big annual holiday is put to bed, the timer upstairs is thinking ahead to the next one. Usually, it's Continental Europe, France in particular, and it's nearly always in a car.

For a food-junkie, driving in the car is probably more significant than I let on. Driving to work, as most people do at least once in a lifetime, I, like everybody else who's had to run the Indian trek along the M50 to get nearly anywhere in Dublin, has either had to avoid or to experience the American statistic that claims that 30 percent of state-siders eat, drink and sleep in their cars.

That's not to say that I want to explain this obsession and everything about my holidays psychologically, because, like food, driving means a lot more to me than just some time out of circulation. Primarily, I just love the anonymity of driving on the wrong side of the road, going somewhere into the unknown, really getting away from it – *it* being my life – and allowing myself happily to forget about what's happening at home. It's something that's always appealed to me: just me and the wifely conscience, going at our own speed, often with a simple plan that's set north or south, or into the unknown. It's like *Pauly Through the Looking Glass*. With such an outlook, we've often arrived in the weirdest of places at crazy hours of the night looking for accommodation and the all-important evening meal.

This approach has not been without its hiccups. *Hiccups* being another colloquialism for 'Where's the food?' For instance, we once arrived in Chauvigny, a medieval market town in the Vienne in western France where five ruined castles guard the various approaches to the citadel, and rambled up to the old town after a long day's driving, with hunger pangs that could be heard in Darfur. Chauvigny's old town is a bit like Bunratty, expect it's not served with traffic or the fuss of Irish dancing, and it's much warmer and more comfortable outdoors. On this occasion, in the state we were in, we made a beeline for what looked like the best restaurant in the village: the one with a really attractive sky-lit dining area under some trees in the main square. Unfortunately, it was also the one that had only a table for two just inside a busy door, with enough traffic to give you a chill and an earache. So, with the wife's casting vote, we declined – to put the kibosh on the enormous *steak frites* that most of the other men in the restaurant seemed to know was good for them. Yes, the lonely, all-powerful voice of womanhood – the Conscience – had a problem with the seating arrangements, the loudness of the staff and, more importantly, how I was leering at the *steak frites* that was been served to a bloke with big eyes and a pointy head, dressed in a yellow-and-red tank top that was at least two sizes too big for him. It didn't matter that he looked like a Teletubby on holiday; I admired him because he was eating what could have been my dinner.

Anyway, we said 'Thanks, but no thanks' and pottered ominously down the hill to a less-populated restaurant, where, sitting
on a two-tabled terrace under some shaded pines, we ordered
apéritifs maisons while we scoured the menu for something whole-
some. The *apéritifs maisons* arrived in plain wooden cups with a
moderate bit of gold bling that had me thinking it was the handi-
work of a humble carpenter. Voices in my head, and particularly
from a First Crusade knight from the Canyon of the Crescent
Moon (read your Indiana Jones), immediately warned me: 'If you
wish for the Grail' – which in my case was *steak frites* – 'drink
wisely, because a false Grail will take them away.' And take them
away it did. By the first taste of the *apéritif maison*, I'd realised our
mistake. The drink was a form of mead, possibly a *chouchen*, the
mead-like drink popular in Brittany, where the fermentation normally involves a mixture of seawater, fresh water and honey. Or
even a badly made Pineau des Charentes, more typical of the area,
made from a blend of unfermented grape must and Cognac,
which in this case seemed to be swimming in overly alcoholic
honeyed herbs. However, by the second gulp, I could taste
enough salt to set up my own Atlantic marine. *Jesus,* I thought, *I'm
drinking seawater.*

The impulse to leave immediately was mitigated by the need
to eat, and the realisation that if it wasn't going to be here, it
wasn't going to be anywhere at all. So we ordered a plate each.
Needless to say, this type of establishment (more Bunrattyian than
Bunratty itself), with its pretensions of chivalry, didn't feel that
steak frites fitted in with what your average knight, or the Duke of
Bedford, for instance, might have felt like eating before he went
out to burn Jeanne d'Arc at the stake. It seemed that there was
definitely a suspicion that the mission statement in this particular
restaurant was boiled down to the maxim that if it couldn't be
caught, it couldn't be cooked.

As always, the Conscience was really happy with her meal, a
fairly decent omelette and a well-balanced salad. My meal, on the
other hand, was a disaster: the house speciality of 'cold chicken
on the bone' with a few salad leaves was only useful if you were
James Bond and you wanted something to hide a piece of micro-
film under with an explanation for, say, what someone did back

in Drumcondra with the £30,000 – do I hear any higher bids? – for the most famous renovation project in history. *Christ, I thought, is this how far civilisation has come? Cold chicken.* And it wasn't just cold, it was refrigerated cold, with enough ice to put on a waiter's face, if you felt the urge to drive your fist through it, like I did. It reminded me of a typical 1980s dinner: leftovers you might have had when, journeying back and forth to the fridge with nothing to do, just picking. It was the type of food you'd give to someone with malaria to lower their temperature. Anyway, it put me in foul humour, and right off my dinner (I use the word loosely), which takes some doing.

As if events couldn't get any worse, the waiter, who, thinking we were English and possibly euro-stupid – the new currency had just been introduced – tried to rob us by diddling us out of our change. In most situations I would let it go, but not for cold chicken.

So, leaving my seat on the loneliest terrace in Christendom, I followed the steward into the restaurant for a row on the merits of dining service, the establishment's obsession with cold chicken, and his bloody good reasons for robbing us. That's all very good, provided you go into battle with some sort of weapon; in this case, a proper understanding of native swearing and the codes and ethics of restaurant complaining. While my French isn't what you'd call bad, the mead had played havoc with my vocabulary, and my phrasebook, like most in the genre, was absolutely useless in the circumstances. When you really want to say, 'You robbed us, you bastard', the words just aren't there, and I just ended up mumbling something in neither French nor English that gave me the bit of confidence to speak a little louder along the lines of *'Mon poulet est froid'*. The waiter, of course, asked me to repeat what I'd said. Angrily, I screamed at him *'Mon poulet est froid'*, not just once but possibly five times, eager to make myself heard, and to impress him, standing smugly in the doorway of a busy kitchen in an empty restaurant. Startled by my obvious anger, the waiter, after a consultation with a manager of sorts, deducted the chicken from the bill, and reimbursed me for a terrible meal, sidestepping the fact that he knew that I knew that he had just robbed me – a fact lost on the manager, who just thought I was an angry fat bloke not sophisticated enough to appreciate cold chicken.

That's all getting away from the day before the first day of the annual holiday, however, the day I'd being anticipating for a full eleven months, since we returned from our last holiday. Taking a month out of our lives in Ireland, nearly every year since the Conscience and I were married, is the real bliss of companionship and love. Getting away from listening to the whining and moaning of *Morning Ireland*, the doom and longevity of Dublin city traffic and all recognisable structures of identity that make us Irish, is like taking a vacation from your life, walking through one of life's few looking glasses into a different world.

Is there a price to pay for this indulgence? Yes, it's called packing. Getting the packing right for four weeks of independence in the old jalopy is an art-form in itself, and a skill only a peculiar genius is capable of. Luckily, this is a chore well suited to the Conscience. If she had been responsible for the invasion of Sicily or the D-Day landing, the Allies would have arrived two days earlier, with twice as much equipment. Her attention to detail and style when it comes to fitting out a car for a road-trip is the stuff of legend. Once, on a meander down through France into Spain for a camping holiday, she managed to fit seventeen tables into a car only half the size of our current jalopy. Seventeen tables? Yes, seventeen. One for the holiday dining table, another for the cooker, another for the utensils, and the rest for our drinking water, washing-up water, lights, books and everything else. In fact, that was the trip when we said we would never camp again.

It was to be strictly a camping holiday, with the usual two visits to vineyards: one on the way down through France and one on the way back up. It didn't work out that way. There was so little room in the car that I couldn't see anything through my rearview mirror, and because we hadn't got air-conditioning in the car, we used to roll down the windows and lean forward together to allow the air to generate a bit of a breeze behind us. Try it, it works fantastically.

We were camping in northern Spain in what was once our favourite four-star campsite. Although it's a fairly large concern by the sea, I won't give you the name for reasons that will become evident below. It has all the amenities of a modern campsite: bar, restaurant, pool, entertainment, supermarket, newsagent and good washing areas. We've gone there on numerous occasions and often lost ourselves in the mêlée of Spanish, German and Dutch tourists. For years, the English language had little currency except in the newsagent, where, peculiarly, they always had one, and only one, copy of the *Guardian* newspaper (the European edition). No matter what time of the year we arrived, I could be guaranteed that that paper would have my name on it. In more recent years, my wife and I noticed a change, when the site seemed to be increasingly hijacked by football-shirt- and skirt-wearing *Ant and Dec's Saturday Night Takeaway* types. In fact, it amazes me sometimes how little clothing you need to fit a George's Cross on – but then again this is a sure sign of the dangers of television's impact on children. *Blue Peter* has a lot to answer for. 'Take one George's Cross and a tea cloth. Today, children, we're going to make an England jersey . . . '

Other flags and emblems flew from tents and caravans on various sections of the campsite. Agincourt and Brighton Pier combined within the confines of another Little England. All we needed was Pinkie. My regular holiday paper wasn't even safe. Going down one afternoon to collect my little nugget of early-evening reading, I was flabbergasted to find that the paper wasn't there. Piecing together some Spanish catchphrases, I nervously enquired whether my paper had arrived. Apparently it had, and apparently it had been sold. What? It can't have been! There's nobody else here likely to buy it. I suspected Pinkie. The following day, I went down five minutes before the papers were due to arrive and loitered, hoping to outwit my faceless adversary, who had potentially ruined my regular holiday haunt. When the papers arrived, I covetously marched the *Guardian* to the counter and paid for it. As I left the shop, I heard the squeakiest of voices ask for the paper. Looking back, I could see a Miss Marple-like elderly lady dressed rather peculiarly; more for a winter fete than for the high-twenties-centigrade heat. On my return to our pitch, my wife suggested that I make contact with the octogenarian and offer her the paper after I'd finished with it. An unlikely scenario. It was time to move on.

The following morning, out on a walk around the campsite, my wife and I decided that we were tired of camping, tired of the noise that the new colours generated, and particularly tired after missing another night's sleep because our wonderfully expensive Hoover Dam-like air-bed camp mattress had decided to take a leak during the night, in the process acquainting us with some of the harder layers of Spanish rock. If that wasn't enough, our two (yes, we brought two on holidays – prepared, or what) even more lavishly expensive quick air pumps (one of which was an electrical gizmo which promised double-fast inflation and deflation times), in sympathy, decided to break down as well. Any number of gods were clearly against us. We took this as an omen. Our days camping could be numbered alongside David Beckham's sell-by date. Anyone keen to embrace the camping should sign up for a Key Camp, or whatever. It's a difficult and tense operation moving tent, sleeping bags, air mattresses and pumps (when they work), mobile kitchen, cooker, seventeen tables and all the various other cooking utensils on an approximately 2,500-mile round trip (not included the boat trip), if you've decided that Spain is where you want to go.

So we returned to our little tent on the plateau, which had been home for a number of holidays, packed our belongings, paid our outstanding bill, and prepared to leave. There was, however, a problem. Our tent. Unlikely ever to camp again, certainly not in this lifetime, we contemplated leaving it where it was. The Conscience made an impassioned plea on behalf of her brother, who could do with a tent. My argument was more persuasive. If he wants it, he can come and get it. And so we left it behind, after carefully removing the tag, which identified a well-known camping shop in Dublin. Other Jonahs to fall that day included another table we'd bought in Saumur which had never worked, and our aforementioned mattress and pumps. We laughed our heads off waving to our erstwhile neighbours, who called after us in a plethora of European tones and languages 'Out for the day?' and 'See you later' as we sniggered back, to ourselves, 'Not unless you're planning a trip to Ireland.' If we regretted anything about our decision, it was that we weren't mosquitoes on the walls of the surrounding tents, when our day out turned into days, then weeks. Did I mention the mosquitoes? No, better leave that for another day. Did the campsite owners hold a grudge? Apparently not. We still get Christmas cards and lavish cylinder-rolled dunce hat-like calendars with the campsite logo emblazoned on the side.

Getting back to the Conscience: if they were chucking out university laurels, myrtles or oak-leaves in car-packing, she would surely be entitled to one of those honorary doctorates. Or even *carruca sarcina egregia cum laude* (car-packing deserving of outstanding praise). Either way, it's something I avoid completely. While she empties the presses of the salad spinner, salt and pepper shakers, knives and forks, bottle openers, teacloths, glasses, cups, picnic basket and mugs, and compartmentalises everything into easy-to-handle bundles or boxes; then washes, tumble-dries and irons every last stitch of clothing that we both possess and that actually fits me; and then 'lovingly' – her word – organises everything neatly in suitcases, suit-bags and kitbags; and finally gets a handle on a month's supply of cosmetics, make-up and toothpaste, I make myself scarce cleaning the car, organising the maps, making the final reading selections for the holiday entertainment, and sorting out my toilet bag. My part in this pre-holiday collaboration usually takes about ten minutes, while I wait desperately out of harm's way for the wife to tell me where to put everything after she's made the all-important choices; a workload that takes her about sixteen hours. I may as well be the taxi driver fiddling with the mirror, wondering should I strike a fare in advance, since I'm going outside the county boundary, or would I be better just not worrying myself to death and letting it happen on the meter. Whatever happens, everywhere else in the house is chaotic. You could cut the tension with a lollipop (if you could find one in the chaos); it's easy to sit there on the sitting-room sofa, building up a hunger, and then just skiving out and getting a snack box while the wife's doing the divil to get us ready.

Every year it's the same. The day before, I'm probably just as busy, and getting a moment to pig out is usually a major worry, what with signing up the holiday and car insurance, filling up the petrol tank, and giving the jalopy the annual tyre check; mind-numbing work that can take all day. In fact, pumping up the tyres for these sorts of trips can be the death of you. For instance, finding a petrol station where the air cylinder is working, in particular, can be a nightmare, and this year was no different. Having pulled into five petrol stations where the air gun was as useless as a catapult facing the might of the Taliban, I finally found one where the thing actually worked. However, as usual when I'm trying to get ahead of myself, I pushed the nozzle on the air hose too aggressively at the tyre valve – on the driver's side. Bang. The air rocketed out of the side of the tyre in a slow lazy hiss that, if you were small enough would have put you to sleep. *Mother of Jaysus*, I said to myself. *How was I so careless?* Realising I'd no room to change the tyre in the station, I drove the car the short distance up a slight hill onto a tarmacadamed surface outside a car salesroom. There I started to wind up the worst jack in living memory, which looked as if it had last seen service in the 1960s somewhere in a tin-pot eastern European republic. By the time I'd the jack pumped up and the tyre off, I had the pox of a misfortune to realise that not only had I fucked up one valve in my haste but that a second value on a tyre on the same side of the car had decided to blow, and was already on its side kissing the surface. *The Lord Jesus*, I thought, *staring up at a blue sky, does anybody up there love me?*

Just as I imagined it couldn't get any worse, the bollox of a jack gave way, and only for a quick-thinking dive that burst the arse in my trousers, the wheel hub, obviously without the wheel, nearly hit the ground, almost ruining any chance of a holiday in France the following day. So, holding on to the side of the car like some overweight four-legged Ichthyostega and trying to keep our only means of transport to France balanced, and at the same time trying desperately to manoeuvre the tyre I had taken off the car and the spare tyre that was beside it nearer to me by using my feet, hoping for my dear life that the cars that were driving by wouldn't drive over my legs, all I needed was my mobile to ring – which, naturally, it did.

It was the Conscience. 'Hi dear, just ringing to see if everything's all right?'

'No, it bloody well isn't, get up here as fast as you can, or else we'll be going nowhere tomorrow.'

Women in these situations are never good. No, I don't need the brother-in-law. No, I don't need AA Rescue. No, I don't need a personality. I just need somebody to help me hold the car up so I can get the bastard set of tyres under the car and the car to safety. But no, it's only rattle, rattle, rattle.

By the time she'd arrived in her white Honda Civic, the little dinky that every car thief in Dublin has tried to rob – the one with the driver's door buckled from idiots trying to break in the door panel through the window rubber – I'd managed to drag the tyres to safety, propped up the car, and asked the manager of the car salesroom for a loan of a proper jack, some air and two of his car-cleaners, who obliged me no end by holding up the car. The most expensive thing about the Civic is probably my wife's sunglasses, although, to be fair, the old Honda is one of life's great survivors.

Despite the numerous attempts on its life, it has only ever encountered one Garda in its lifetime. That was once, around seven o'clock one morning, when a Ban Garda pointed out to us as we left for work that the car wasn't taxed. Once in six years – and it was probably three weeks overdue at the time. Far more vigilant are the yobbos who keep knocking on the door, particularly around dinner time, when I'm trying to make chips on the sly, asking: 'Hey, mister, you haven't taxed your Honda Civic – is it for sale?' Despite this interest, we've always said 'No, it's only a runaround, and anyway there's no power in it.' But they still call, religiously, once every couple of months.

Once when, incidentically, we'd just arrived home from France, after being away for a month, friends called, and I had to go up to the local supermarket to stock up on a few provisions. This was the day, I was sure, the Guards would call. Driving by the local fast-food drive-through, I let a car reverse in ahead of me – a car in which three of the occupants subsequently put on monkey hats. In a hurry, and hungry, I didn't give it a moment's thought until I was driving past the drive-through again, on the way out, having done my supermarket shopping – by which time there were Guards everywhere. Realising that, yes, the three blokes with the monkey helmets had probably robbed the restaurant, I stopped to tell the Guards: 'I saw everything, and if you want a full description of the gang, call to my address in half an hour, after my dinner.' Looking back, they must have thought I was out of my mind. Needless to say, I'm still waiting for them to call.

Anyway, getting back to this year's trip to France, having fallen asleep watching the Conscience do all the work packing the car, I was at least refreshed the following morning to start the car and finally begin the first leg of the summer holidays: the mad dash to Cork for the ferry to Roscoff. It's worked for us for a number of years, whether we've camped in the Loire, Gascony or the Savoie, venturing over the border into Spain on the odd occasion, or hired villas, gîtes or mobile homes in Provence or the Dordogne. Taking to the roads, often with no plan, has been equally enjoyable; driving on one particular day, obsessionally, you could say, following the sun from Italy through France to Spain. Stopping in a town because it happens to be on the way to nowhere is a great way to holiday and is much better, in our opinion, than the itinerary of always having to be somewhere, and by a certain time. Mostly, however, we have stopped in France, getting stuck into the food, the wine and the anonymity.

From a fat bloke's perspective, it has always meant, unbelievably, weight loss, whether from drinking more water than normal – because of the warmer weather – or eating far more salads. Or maybe it's because for a month the Conscience is watching every morsel I put into my mouth, running security checks on my diet and policing what's good or isn't good for me.

Anyway, having been up all night doing the bejaysus for what is usually a 2,500-mile drive, we normally aim to be out of Dublin before noon if we're planning to make the four o'clock sailing from Rosslare. On this occasion, we had planned to be on the road by 11 AM, knowing that we were driving to Cork for the 5 PM sailing to Roscoff. However, by 12.15, we're stuck on the M50 southbound.The car only inches forward, and anxiety levels in the car slowly rise to breaking point. The wife makes one of those 'We're not going to make it' stares at me, unable to verbalise the trauma that's filling the valley between my seat and hers. It's a stare I've experienced twice before, on both occasions when going with Irish Ferries from Rosslare to Cherbourg, in the days when they didn't run a low-cost service.

On the first occasion, we got stuck in the many traffic jams that littered the N11 through Rathnew, Arklow and Gorey. Eventually, at 3.40 PM, and about twenty minutes from Rosslare, for a 4 o'clock sailing, we rang Irish Ferries and asked them would the ship be delayed for any reason. 'No,' they said, 'we sail at 4 PM.' Now, according to our ticket, we were supposed to check in half an hour before sailing, so technically we had defaulted, but hey, this is Ireland, and bureaucracy often hangs from a skipping rope. On the one hand, you're worrying yourself sick that you're going to miss the sailing, while at the same time some ancestral whisper is telling you: *Don't worry, they'll wait for you.* So, we rang them back: 'Is there any chance you could possibly wait for us, we'll be there in five minutes?' (A lie – but worth a punt.) 'Well, we can't promise anything, but get here as fast as you can. The final decision will be the captain's.' Ramming the bejaysus out of the accelerator, we tried our best to make it there for 4 o'clock, and on the button of 4 PM we arrived at the port. 'Do you know what time it is?' asks the clerk in the hut. 'We do.' 'Oh, you do, do you. Well, I'll have to ask the captain.' Grand. A phone call later, the reply: 'He says you're lucky. Go on, but hurry up.' Which we did, driving into the ship under the hundreds of people on the top-deck looking down on us fools, collectively lifting their eyes to heaven, because we were the ones who would ensure that the boat would probably miss the tide and arrive in France an hour or two later than expected.

Taken in isolation, this mightn't seem like an extraordinary story, until you realise that we went through the same ordeal the following year, once again driving under the hundreds of people on the top deck looking down on us fools, and collectively lifting their eyes to heaven.

So, stuck as we are on the M50, this time going to Cork, the fact that I could have done a bit more to get us down faster starts to come between the Conscience and myself. 'This is your fault. We're going to miss that sailing. What time is the sailing? Five o'clock? We'll never make it.' And so we plod on, finally leaving Naas behind us at 2 PM, with a potential three-hour journey ahead of us, not forgetting that this takes no consideration of the fact that we are again requested to check in at least half an hour before departure. With the original plan to stop somewhere for a bit of grub along the way gone out the window, the car is a hungry place to be. Further delays in and around Cashel, Mitchelstown and Fermoy leave us in a predicament we are experiencing for the third time. By the time we reach the ferry port, I'm fading away with hunger, worry and tension. Luckily, there's a queue of cars waiting to get on board, and our concerns evaporate.

Once settled into our cabin, five-odd hours without food began to take its toll, and we quickly made our way to the restaurant before I hyperventilated. After dinner, we treated ourselves to some champagne – consolation for missing dinner during the day – with friends in the bar, which resulted in a later-than-anticipated start the following morning. Exiting on the sunny shores of Roscoff in Brittany with a slight hangover fuelled a desperate need for carbohydrates. Our original plan was to head south immediately, but driving below par and a little slower than usual, a dash across France's most westerly peninsula for a decent spot of Sunday lunch (*avec,* thankfully, *steak frites*) in a favourite spot – Saumur in the Loire Valley – seemed a much better option. It was a Sunday morning coming down and I couldn't get food into my body fast enough. The sun shone and the cure flowed.

Three days later, we were in a hotel in Carjac further south, passing a few spare days before we were due to arrive in Provence, where we'd hired a villa; a different experience for us from our usual escapades. In the hotel room, each of us relaxing over a book, our little bit of heaven was disturbed by noisy voices, bellowing up from the hotel restaurant's terrace below, which doubled as a breakfast and dining area. Usually, the voices, in such out-of-the-way hotels as this one, at this time of the year, are mostly French, soft – the school term not yet over – and a mixture of mid-week business language, which never rises a decibel above a heated hush, and the elderly whispers of the semi-retired tourists. And then, of course, there are the oddities like us.

On this occasion, late in the afternoon, the waiting staff, making a minimum of fuss setting the tables for the evening service – putting out the cutlery, plates and glasses – were upstaged like intrusive whistles in a library of peace, and, of course, the voices were Anglo-Saxon, and American in particular. Earlier, the American kids had loudly interrupted my morning's reading – Simon Schama's take on the French Revolution, *Citizens*. *How bloody appropriate*, I thought to myself, as I wrestled with the heat and the mosquito bites on my ankle. So loud, intensive and annoying were the Brash Street Kids that it caused a slight row between the wife and myself. We got so boisterous that I expected some little over-fussy administrative functionary to walk into our room, stare out from our curtains and announce, like Duc de la Rochefoucauld-Liancourt on 15 July 1789 to Louis XVI: 'Sire, this is not a riot, it is a revolution.'

By dinner time, the noise levels had returned to normal, and the kitchen smells coming from below were feeding my appetite. Sitting in my underpants, admiring my figure – when I bent a certain way, it gave the impression that I had lost some weight – I enjoyed with the Conscience a half-bottle of sparkling wine we'd bought in the Loire Valley three days earlier. It was really cold and refreshing, and much cheaper than the restaurant's apéritif. You might wonder how in the name of jaysus we were able to keep champagne cold in this weather. Well, it was easy. We'd emptied the hotel's mini-bar selection and filled it up with our own half-bottles of sparkle. We also had our own fridge – yes, we always bring our mini-fridge on holidays – filled with a regular supply, in case of emergencies. Not surprisingly, we are always the ones in any hotel we stay in who are constantly asking for more ice.

Dressing myself for dinner, the delusion of thinking that I'd lost weight was dashed by the obvious discomfort I experienced when I stretched my clobber against my bulging body. Sun, rain or snow, the clothes always betray you, even if your eyes see differently. Jesus, I thought, if I could only go around in the nip all day, I'd never worry about putting on weight. And I'm convinced I look slimmer in the nip than I do in my clobber.

Anyway, before I could get too philosophical, the dinner bell went berserk in my head, and before I could say 'I'll have the *steak frites*', we were hovering over our menus and listening in on the Americans, who had decided that they were going to tell the whole restaurant their life story, as if we were camping up on Walton's Mountain and John-Boy and Marie-Ellen were the only storytellers in town and it was only a mo before they'd wish us goodnight.

They're from New Orleans, the engineer-cum-businessman father is Atticus Finch, and an all-round wise-owl to his children – who incidentally bear no resemblance to Scout and Jem – and his wife has a whining voice. The youngest child is a wannabe Roman historian who just has to tell you in triplicate everything clever about himself. He's the type of kid you want to frighten with stories of Attila the Hun and every other bogeymen. The parents, of course, indulge their kids in that typically American way, so much so that the family take their 'summer vacation' to coincide with their kid's historical fantasies. So they've been to Italy and Wales for the Romans – Wales of course being the birthplace of Roman civilisation, according to the hotel's pint-size Cicero. His father tells us that his son did remarkably well in a recent school report on – guess what – the Romans; this qualification is seemingly enough to justify boring the other guests for the next hour and a half on the history of the Romans in Europe, in English, as if we're all foreigners and, really, these dudes were dangerous dudes who ruled, guess what, Europe. Oh yeah, I say to myself, I've heard of that place. Maybe it's because I was born here forty-odd years ago and have lived here ever since. Thankfully – and we are reassured of this by Junior Cicero in case we weren't aware of it – yes, the Romans unfortunately didn't make it to America. Well, fuck me.

The Americans make no effort to speak French, ordering everything in English and being so stupid as to ask the waiters difficult questions about the mechanics of cooking. What does *flétan* mean? It's halibut? Hali-who? *Poisson*, fish. What type of fish? Flatfish? Is it Californian? No, French. How is it cooked? And so it goes on, as if we're sitting in a fish restaurant in Milwaukee and the waiter, when not desperately hoarding his tips to get him through college, has taken time off from giving grinds on marine biology to Jacques-Yves Cousteau.

And just when you think it's time to reflect on the falling night sky in Carjac and the subtle whistling of the birds, besides the multitude of mosquitoes which are feeding on my ankles, Son Number 2 lets it be known that he's a student of the Greeks, and off he meanders, boring the assembled Francophiles and, in particular, a married couple from Reading who happen to be civil servants and sitting nearest the epicentre, on Troy, Achilles, Hector and Priam. *Priam?* I say to myself. Surely this kid is reading from a script. I wonder if they're a travelling troupe, pygmy in origin, who are playing 'Guess Who?' with the Carjac homeboys. Straining my neck like a boa constrictor doing contorted impressions of a manila rope, I finally glimpse the Brady Bunch. Jesus, I say to myself, the kid looks like Mats Wilander's little brother, except that he and his family are obviously not Swedish.

The history lessons continues apace with Cicero and his bigger brother, who has a mouth to rival Herodotus, offering opening statements, main arguments and closing speeches for junior president. The local-authority civil servant from Reading, who with his wife has been politely playing audience to the historical racket, minding his own business and generally congratulating Jor-El and Lara on their Kryptonite double-act and saying how wonderful it is to have such bright, intelligent progeny at their feet, suddenly finds himself embarrassed. Père Brady in his know-all so-what-do-you-do? tone questions the lowly career bureaucrat on middle-England's transportation nuts and bolts.

OK, so there's a natural inquisitiveness to know your name and where you're from: it's friendly, passes a bit of time and, what the hell, it's nice to be nice. Then the questions get a little too intrusive for my liking and, by the look of the bloke from Reading, too intrusive for his liking too. What's with the third degree? Didn't he tell you his name, where he's from, even what he did for a living? No, that wasn't good enough for you. You had to throw him a curve ball, Mr Bloody Almighty Know-all. What's with you Americans? I start to chew more bread, grinding it in my teeth like I'm biting through the rope that's supposed to restrain me, as if an army surgeon is struggling to remove a bullet from my hole. Feeling myself turning green with rage, my fat bloke emerges, with some Hulk-like anger. I'm close to butting in and saying something I'll later regret, until my wife gives me the look, the Conscience at work, you know, the rhyming little head-bob that trips out the usual: 'You can take the fat bloke away from the anger but you can never take the anger away from the fat bloke.'

Not waiting for an answer, Père Brady tells us of his own predicament, alluding to the fact that CNN – apparently the only news channel in the world – got it all wrong, and that rich people also suffered a few years ago during Hurricane Katrina, and how his engineering works had a bit of a meltdown, how he split from his partner, how he continued to pay his staff a salary out of his confirmation money and retained them, by golly, even though there was no work in the Big Easy, and how a tree in their garden fell on their neighbour's house. All major, traumatic events – I was particularly upset for the poor unfortunate who probably now lived in a tree house next door to the family from hell – but not enough to have most people in the restaurant, and certainly those with American English and within listening range, crying into their candle-lit brandies. And certainly not when Père Brady overestimated the Reading civil servant's position and started popping questions on railway procurement, the steel crisis and advances in civil engineering. Of course, the man from Reading should never have told us – we were all listening at this stage – that he was involved in the finance department of the local authority, but especially not the American, who presumed that the civil servant was buying trains, planes and automobiles, when any eejit could have told him that the bloke from Reading just sat in the corner of the open-plan office at a tidy desk with the coffee cup stamped 'Dad' and that his position in the finance depart-ment was accounting for pens, paper and envelopes.

During the course of my meal, I realised that I tend to eat more when I'm angry, particularly bread, which the waiters keep replenishing as soon as I've made my way through another slice. I'm not so much your butter-on-bread type of bloke. For me, bread is more about the prelude to a feed, or the soggy cushion for mopping up the French sauces. And on the subject of waiters, the guy serving at our table was a ringer for Harpo Marx, with the weirdest thatch of bright yellow hair you've ever seen. Mind you, apart from the hair and the lost-boy looks, the waiter was as sullen as you could get, the type with understandably no English, who is so angry that tourists visit his country that he's unable to speak or smile. I wanted to ask him, on a scale of one to ten, how much did he hate the Brady Bunch?

The following night, we found ourselves pitched opposite the Bradys and, as you'd expect, after the introductions and small talk about where we're from, Père Brady popped the question: 'So, Paul, what do you do?' Expecting the ambush, I'd already grabbed the biggest piece of bread on my plate and shoved it into my mouth. My guttural retort was, as I had planned, an incoherent mumble. However, the big bold American asked again, while I poked and pointed to my big, fat, bulging mouth. By the time my embarrassed wife told him what I did, the American had made up his mind. Looking across at the little Irishman with the squirrel cheeks, I could see that he knew he was dealing with a glutton of sorts. The general bestiality of the encounter was reinforced when, moments later, Harpo Marx gestured towards our menu and awaited our order. Unable to clear my gob fast enough, I had to point at the menu. At this stage, the waiter had also made up his mind about me – 'Why can't these bloody tourists learn our language?' – which was the same argument I'd been making to my wife about the Americans for two days.

By the end of the week, we'd arrived in Lambesc, near Aix, where we'd hired a villa for two weeks. I had planned to use the swimming pool and gardens to train, and to make some decent inroads into my mountain of fat over the next fortnight. To make my training camp – boot camp, if you will – interesting, I decided to go the whole hog and bring my old football boots – the still impressive-sounding Predators – in which I'd scored hundreds of goals both ten years ago and, since, in my dreams. As my old leather football had long since hung up its own boots, I went and bought a new leather football the week before we left. Obviously, I'd paid over the odds for the football, but I didn't care, when I thought it would be blissful soloing up and down the Provençal back garden, adding a bit of cardiovascular training to the swimming regime. However, when we arrived, the weather was in the high thirties, and it was much too warm even to sit in the sun. I did try. I went out at about seven o'clock one morning and ran up and down the garden about five times, doing my best Jimmy Keaveney before giving up in a lather of sweat, absolutely knackered. As the morning got warmer, thoughts of running, or even walking, became more and more ludicrous, and so I decided to put my feet up and watch a bit of the World Cup and a couple of old James Bond films on the television, though it's not quite the same to hear Sean Connery say in his best James Bond: *'Je m'appelle Bond, James Bond.'*

Late that afternoon, I went out to the pool to do a few lengths. It was still warm but manageable – if you could dodge the various flies, bees and dragonflies, who seem to think they've hired the villa for the fortnight and have decided it's even too warm for them to bother to go hunting breadcrumbs, fruit, pollen or other micro-flies, and so have congregated around the pool. Without getting myself wet, the only exercise I did by the pool for half an hour was dredging it, clearing what it seems a little foolish to call foreign objects. Nevertheless, it had to be done. Despite building up a bit of an appetite, the last thing I wanted to happen – if I ever got the chance to exercise – was to swallow someone else's dinner.

Anyway, no sooner had I cleared the pool than I had to do it again. And again. *Jesus,* I thought, *I'm being exercised by flies. I wouldn't find myself working this hard watching a Jane Fonda Workout video. If I'm not careful, I could end up spending the whole holiday going back and forth to the pool house, cleaning away the flies and wasps and not even getting a swim.*

I tried screaming: 'Get the fuck out of my swimming pool!' Nothing. I tried again: 'Get the fuck out of my swimming pool!' Again, nothing.

Then the Conscience woke up. I'd forgotten she was asleep on the veranda. 'Why the hell are you shouting? Are you out of your mind?'

'It's the poxy flies – they won't get out of the pool. I'm sick of them. What am I supposed to do?'

'Grow up, will you. They're only flies. You just have to put up with them. And you'll solve nothing by losing the head.'

That's the Conscience for you, I thought. Never takes my side, even against flies.

As I walk around the pool, deranged, the wife gradually goes back to sleep. The monotony of walking in rectangles makes me tired, and I decide it's about time I blew up the his and hers lilos that we've brought all the way from Ireland. It takes ages, blowing and huffing, but I finally manage it, although it takes every bit of breath away from me. It's getting worse: I'm now being exercised by inanimate objects. I feel like an exhibit in a museum, with the director sticking pins in a plastic doll that looks just like me. I want to lie down and sleep forever, and now I'm going to get my chance – on a piece of rubber three feet by six, hopefully floating backwards and forwards across the pool, having a bit of me-time. However, as usual, the gods are against me, and it doesn't quite work out that way. The problem is that I'm just a bloody big fat bloke, and rolling on to a lilo supported by five feet of water isn't something that comes naturally to me.

You'd think that jumping up and staying on a see-through piece of plastic would be easy. Well, it's not. Each time I try to swing my legs across the rubber mattress, to, as they say, 'get up on it', I fall off the other side. I try again. And again. And again. Each time I try a different approach. From the bottom upwards, almost walking up it, doesn't work. Diving from the side of the pool on top of it doesn't work. Waking up the wife and getting her to hold it straight doesn't work. Rolling over on top of it from the side of the pool doesn't work. Getting up on it arse-first doesn't work. No matter which way I try it, it doesn't work. Not that I give up. No way. The bloody set of lilos cost the price of a small package holiday, and there's no way they are going to get the better of me. We'd bought them about three years before in Gordes, a small, picturesque hilltop village in Provence, over the valley from Roussillon, where Beckett famously played hide-and-seek with the Germans during World War II. Who in their right minds buys two lilos up the side of a mountain? In fact, what sort of a madman would open a shop so far above sea level that only sells marine equipment? Next time you're in the area, go in and see him, and while you're at it, ask him how in the name of jaysus a fat bloke is meant to get up on the lilos he sells.

By the time the dinner bell in my brain is ringing six o'clock, the gods grant me some success. Finally, doing something I can't remember, I manage to stay up. I don't get off to bask in my glory – and spend the rest of the afternoon trying to figure out how I'd done it.

The wife has been up on her lilo for two hours, and has gone for at least three naps. Lying on my throne, it dawns on me how much water I've splashed out of the pool. The water mark on the pool is down a foot, and the patio around it looks like Ringsend every couple of years, when the tide comes in with a vengeance. But it's no rest for the wicked; it's nibble time, and before I get a chance to get a well-deserved rest, I'm in the kitchen searching out the goodies.

Nibbles are deadly when it comes to putting on the holiday fat, so I try to keep on the better side of moderation – not that I could ever say I've been victorious in that. The problem is, I just can't say no to trying something different. In the supermarket in France, there's usually a whole big long row devoted to all sorts of nibbles I've never even heard of, and the voices in my brain get uncontrollably excited, encouraging me to buy everything around me. It's like Adam in the Garden, tempted by a thousand Eves. Usually on these trips to the supermarket, the Conscience acts the policeman, holding the snake in check, chasing all the other Eves away, but even then it's not below me to sneak an extra packet down the checkout in between the peppers and the salads when the Conscience isn't looking.

Contemplating my weight problem, I realise that the fat bloke is always last to get his room, last to leave the pool, last to eat and last to find his bed. In fact, he's last to do everything. And in many ways, he's always travelling, carrying the extra suitcase or extra bit of luggage. You can see him in your mind's eye, struggling with everything he does. That man is me, always on the go, always getting nowhere, never getting ahead of anybody else. In fact, I'm completely uneconomical in everything I do, and, not surprisingly, that includes my attitude to food. It's not that just because I'm bigger, slower, and find it harder to get around, I'm probably carrying a little more luggage, not just around my girth but also around my mind: psychological baggage, for want of another phrase. This is all pretty important introspection, particularly as I sit out on the patio eating my first meal of the day and watching a raiding party of magpies flying in low over our hosts' cherry trees. Magpies, you see, have it every which way. No mortgage, no home, no cares, no baggage – just natural-born raiders. And incidentally, when was the last time you saw a fat magpie? Well, forgetting about Malcolm McDonald and Paul Gascoigne, probably never.

Now, looking out into the Provençal morning wouldn't normally remind me of home, but on this occasion it did, because we also have a cherry tree in our back garden. From the start, buying the cherry tree seemed an attractive proposition. Yes, we had a vacancy in our *petit* city garden. Yes, the notion of a cherry tree seemed rather in keeping with the notions we have of ourselves, and yes, the thought of picking our own cherries while sipping an Americano in the evening on our sun-soaked deck was particularly appealing. You get the picture.

So, on a wet July last year, when standing in an even wetter garden centre, we frogmarched the last remaining morello-cherry tree to the checkout. *Me, me, me,* it had shouted to us, the myopic amateur gardeners, who had eyes only for the 'Cherry' label, accepting the 'Morello' addendum on its merits as a brand name or some other fancy additive of distinction. Gagged, with a plastic bag over its head, and tied down in the back seat of our car, the cherry tree, appropriately enough in the circumstances, dripped a few tears of rain as we drove it away.

At home, and once the cherry tree had been ensconced temporarily in a leftover pot that was two sizes too big for it, we read the little elastic-fixed label that hung from the third branch like a joker on the end of a bungee rope: 'Cherry Morello – *prunus cerasus*, from the *subgenus cerasus* (cherry) native to Europe and south-west Asia'. More importantly – and as anyone in the garden centre could have told us if we'd bothered to ask – 'commonly referred to as the Sour Cherry'. Sour in the sense of 'inedible', unless you had a degree in jam-making or the time to rustle up cherry pie.

A quick call to the garden centre confirmed Sod's gardening laws. Yes, of course, they did edible cherry trees, but no, they wouldn't be available until the spring – six months away. Yes, we're very sorry, and no, they don't grow on trees.

Nevertheless, they kindly told us that there were four edible cherry trees: bing, lapin, sam and stella. Of course, this didn't solve the problem with our little specimen, the sour impostor. Christmas came and went, while we built a gallows and continued to plague garden centres about bings, lapins, sams and stellas. It sounds like a who's who at a dodgy jazz club. By spring, amazingly, we'd had a change of heart, when the morello started to show off, rather beguilingly, a magnificent frock of white flowers. And so it was decided that 'Little Mo' was no longer in the family's way and was deemed to have justifiably cheated Madame La Guillotine.

Our cherry-tree obsession brings me nicely to where we are now, in the back garden of the Provençal holiday home we've hired from one of those pretty couples who seem to have everything, in particular a responsible relationship with food and also, in this case, not one but three cherry trees. And, unlike our desperate little so-and-so, their *montmorencys* were all edible – so much so in fact that Madame Bobillier (the joke for the two weeks was that she was married to Bobillier the Builder) told us that we could eat of the trees, if we so desired. Were they bing, lapin, sam or stella? Sadly, our conversational French didn't get past the misunderstanding about a barber-shop quartet.

Anyway, before we had time to do any fancy Adam-and-Eveing, four of the biggest magpies this side of Newcastle seemed to think that the cherry trees were their personal fiefdom and set siege to the thousands of ripe fruit on the trees. Even eating of the fruit liberally, as instructed, we were no match for the bloody magpies, who were working shifts dive-bombing like cherry-crazed Stukas. Not that we didn't use cunning to scare them. No, sir, we tried every trick in the book to outwit what Shakespeare calls in *Macbeth* 'maggot pies'. We even tried the guard-the-tree-with-the-dummy trick, setting up a deckchair under the trees and positioning a rather fetching *Marie Claire* centrepiece photo shoot with numerous French bods, so that, flying in from 250 feet, you might think that pint-size super-models were guarding the trees. Did it work? Did it . . . . The crafty buggers were fooled for a while but were back eating the cherries in the afternoon. I reacted like George Bernard Shaw when he read Chekhov's plays (including, presumably, *The Cherry Orchard*), threatening to rip up my complete oeuvre and writing *Heartbreak House* as a tribute to the Russian master. Having not quite the canon of Mr Shaw, I nevertheless tore up *Marie Claire* and promised to write an allegorical play about the destruction of European civilisation. My publishers, reading this, would probably say: 'Just write the book you promised us first.'

We even hung white flags and bags from the trees – which the magpies took as a flag of surrender. In fact, two days into our holidays, not one piece of tree-fruit remained. By day three, the *pica picas* (scientific name – so bad they named them twice) were gone, and we were left to ponder paradise without fruit, forbidden or otherwise.

As a postscript, I'll jump ahead a little, to when we got back to Dublin from France, three weeks later, when our little morello was already summering its sour cherries. We thought of making a bakewell tart but before we had time to laugh off suggestions that the Provençal rustlers might be migratory, and eager to pay us a visit, we were raided by a well-hung mob of wood pigeons – winged Dick Turpins with grey handkerchiefs up to their beaks – who laid siege to our Little Mo and, within hours, had departed with all our cherries except one. I remember sitting in our small suburban garden with one extremely bitter cherry hanging from the slenderest of threads, blabbering to myself that Lopakhin in *The Cherry Orchard* was wrong when he told Madame Ranevskaya: 'The only remarkable thing about your cherry orchard is its dimensions . . . producing a crop every year which nobody actually wants'. All I can say is: tell that one to the birds.

*

Anyway, our time in Lambesc flew – nearly as fast as the bloody magpies, in fact – and before long, I had swum about twelve lengths of the pool during the course of a fortnight, kicked a football up and down the garden for five minutes and spent twelve eight-hour days killing flies, wasps, mosquitoes and other amphibious insects, who were sharing our pool but not the rent. Like every other adventure in my life, it was another lost opportunity for me to lose weight. Ultimately, the amount of time I'd spent exercising in the south of France was about the same as it would have taken me to train a budgie to say 'You're a muppet'. Anyway, we were on our way to our next destination: a hotel we'd always promised ourselves we'd visit if we were ever in the area. I had a week to blow off a pound or two, at least.

Not that I wasn't feeling like I should have done more. Sitting with my wife on the terrace of the Hostellerie du Domaine de la Reynaude, I saw how the other half live when a fat man with small reading glasses, dressed in matching beige shirt and pants, and with a white bull terrier by his side, stood staring up at our balcony like a stupid gladiator and his mate waiting for the thumbs up (or down) from Caesar and his missus. Instead of the statutory acknowledgment '*Ave Caesar morituri te salutant*', the stupid Frenchman stood to attention, calming the bull terrier with '*Bon bull, bon bull*', with the same intonation that John Hurt uses to mimic Richard Harris in *The Field*. I had just poured us a couple of glasses of cheap champagne and emptied a few olives and other nibbles into a set of bowls but, conscious that we were being watched as we ate, I was embarrassed into abstinence. This went on for three-quarters of an hour, the fella and the dog staring up at us, occasionally complimenting each other, I thought, through growls and guttural '*Bon bull*'s, and we like idiots frozen in our plastic white chairs, unable to look anywhere but down on our stalkers. The man held the passive dog in tow with one of those long pulley-type leads that you could stretch across a race-track as a substitute finishing-line. Every so often, he would yank a little on the lead, irritating his best friend, who had one of those

Staffordshire necks that could drag a cyclist up Alp D'Huez, whether he was on EPO or not. The dog, whose face was angrier than his temperament, would nonchalantly turn his neck ever so slightly in annoyance without shifting his focus from the terrace.

As this surreal Mexican stand-off went on in the sweltering Provençal heat, I was busy looking up phrase books to find the vernacular for 'Do you want something?' or 'A bone, perhaps?', or, better still, while pointing out to the right at the fields of corn, lavender, sunflowers and vines: 'Elysium is that way.' After about an hour, it was irritating me so much that I started to mutter my anger but only managed to annoy my wife. Modern-day Don Quixotes and Sancho Panzas, I thought, standing looking at a fat windmill. I wondered, as the minutes clicked into the next hour, who would be better at tilting at windmills: the master, with his bruising Germanic snout, or the gladiator of the canine race, with his lazy, bow-legged gait? Or, indeed, who was the master and who was the servant? But in a flash, they were gone.

Hostellerie du Domaine de la Reynaude is a couple of kilometres from Aurons, just outside Salons. In previous years, when we'd passed through, it had been booked out. It gave the impression of being a popular destination, away from the hustle and bustle. It had plenty of fields to walk in, and a large pool and tennis courts. However, by the time we got the opportunity to stay there, it was an unmitigated nightmare. To cap it all, it was too bloody warm to do anything. The hotel's restaurant was particularly disappointing – and was not helped by the fact that we'd decided on the *demi-pension*, or the set menu, which started with a buffet, followed by a main course, and then a buffet dessert.

Now, generally speaking, I do badly when offered a buffet. Over the years, I've found it to be an invitation to get stuck in, working the kitchen to overtime, so much so that we've never stayed in such places two nights running, as my exaggerated dining habits come between the wife and myself. In these circumstances, over-indulgence isn't just a problem for the headspace and the Conscience; it primarily affects the stomach and the whole art of digestion. For the normal eater, after proper mastication food sleepwalks the short journey from the oesophagus down to the stomach and finally loop-the-loops through the intestines until a call of nature the following morning tells you that 'You're wanted in the loo'. I have never been a masticator, however, and usually break all comers' records for eating my food by the shovel-full, tractor-like. For me, it's all about speed. Get it into you as fast as you can, before the nerve triggers have time to break wind and press the panic button. It's like building a roundabout around the M50 of satiation and putting in flyovers to motorways that never end. So, no sooner is my food loosely tucked up in the bed of my stomach than it decides that it wants to be read a story, or to be walked around the house with a soother up its arse because I have eaten too much food, far too fast, and not an organ in my body can get to sleep. It's like living with a child in the throes of the terrible twos every day of your life.

The problem is that these memories usually get buried whenever I see 'buffet' on a menu. My first reaction is usually, as I have mentioned in other chapters, Pavlovian: my salivation sensors do cartwheels to catch the attention of some imaginary Ivan Petrovich Pavlov who lurks somewhere under a chef's hat. Then 'the look' kicks in from the Conscience, and I have second thoughts – my wife's facial expression in itself a Pavlovian trigger for all the pain and sleepless nights that are synonymous with the Big B. In other words, when I see 'buffet', I always see pain, eventually.

On this occasion, however, the buffet was small, mostly because we were the last down to dinner and the other guests seemed to have tucked in with relish. We were also going head to head with a wedding party, who, it seemed, had got not only first refusal on the finest food but also the best seats. We, on the other hand, were relegated to what looked like the cheap seats just inside the restaurant's doors, away from the romantic terrace. It was also a bit of a blind spot for waiters coming and going – what you might call a busy junction, which, if it existed in Ireland, wouldn't have got planning permission without traffic lights or a dodgy brown paper envelope. Where we were sitting would have been unpleasant if it was January, never mind in June. Nevertheless, it was dinner time, and we were hungry – although the service was as friendly as dinner hour during the Siege of Stalingrad, with as much chance of copping a sniper's bullet as getting the waitress's attention. When the waitress finally arrived, she was as po-faced as Marshal Konev when Stalin acknowledged that he was giving Marshal Zhukov the honour of capturing the Reichstag and hoisting Soviet colours over Berlin. And I'm sure that the wine waiter, a nasty bit of work in his own right, tried to hit me with the cork.

Anyway, there we were sitting down to our aperitifs – which finally arrived, along with a bottle of ice-cold rosé – waiting our turn to go up and raid the buffet for the starter. The rosé was so chilled that it reminded me of the stories that Baron Philippe de Rothschild of Mouton-fame often served Château d'Yquem – the dog's bollocks of Sauternes – as a sorbet, and I wanted to ask the waitress, waiter or restaurant manager, if I was fast enough to stop one, whether we could have two bowls and spoons for our wine. The thought passed. Having eaten as much as a bulimic monk on retreat – with his jaws wired – during the day, I was really looking forward to a decent dig-in, and my initial buffet negativity had long since been sent to the back of class by the Council of Hunger, who had met in emergency session in my head, deeming that, now, buffets were the greatest invention in the history of the world and that all mankind was eagerly awaiting how I'd measure up to the challenge of eating everything in sight. Temptation was easy: it was helped by the trays of hors d'œuvres, crudités and charcuterie that were been carried by our table on the waiting staff's shoulders like miniature popes.

Such was the traffic from the kitchen to the wedding party, however, that it was only safe to exit the considerably slow lane, where we were seated, into the accident-prone overtaking lane – after half an hour the floor resembled the Hostellerie du Domaine de la Reynaude's players' re-enactment of the H-Block dirty protest, obviously without the blankets – when the number of juggernauts of food, going at full speed, seemed to abate somewhat.

Nevertheless, post-rush-hour, getting to the buffet counter in one piece without a plastering of *soupe à l'oignon fratinée* or *salade de harengs marines au vin blanc* was a little tricky, seated as we were. While we sat half-up, half-down on our seats, like nervous L-drivers making our way down the slip-road of the M50 for the first time, all the other guests, who didn't seem to have a caravan of tray-carriers going by their table, were making their way up for seconds, and I was sure that the bloke with the bulldog was making his way up for a third. Did I mention that there was a bulldog in the restaurant? Oh yes, cometh the man, cometh the dog. And there he was, munching away on what I assumed was my buffet starter, as the legions on the cuisine-shuttle zoomed by our table.

I wouldn't normally be an advocate of junction boxes or traffic lights on a roundabout, and certainly not in a restaurant, but if Jacques Chirac (now of course the former president of France) had walked into the restaurant at that moment with his minister for the environment and both of them had got down on their knees and proceeded to draw a yellow box to the right of our table, I would have given my life to the Foreign Legion as a mark of respect and sold my wife into slavery. Of course, this didn't happen. The Conscience told me to calm down. Her own hunger buds putting appetite before conjecture, we indicated briefly with our hands, and with our backs bent and waving our white napkins like it was Bloody Sunday, we slouched down towards the buffet.

I nearly lost an eye bustling my way through the snipping waiters with their pointy trays, my wife muttering behind me to be careful and not to be so aggressive. 'I'm unarmed,' I protested, to deaf ears. By the time I got to the buffet counter, most of the starters were gone, probably gorged by the canine and his master, who, from the end of the restaurant, I could hear congratulating his pet with loud cries of '*Bon bull!*' This, of course, was winding me up, and I was tempted to fight the *bull* for my dinner. Or, at worst, remembering how Frau Emmy Von N. had told Freud about the boy eating the white mouse, I wondered how bull tasted on a spit.

My wife tried calming me again, pointing out that, while most of the charcuterie, dainty delicacies and fatty nibbles were gone, there were enough lettuces, tomatoes, carrots and dressing to start a green revolution – not the sort of conversation that was likely to appease me, you understand. So how does my wife react? Well, like any true husband-loving Judas would: she accused me of being childish. 'Childish? Is that what I am to you?' I hurled back, my bark like the bulldog's. A glass of wine later, I was calm, the lettuce leaves, tomatoes, tapenade and extra portions of bread having given me a high. Is this how junkies experience it? Lying back in my seat, almost in a different world, the salty earthiness of the black olives coaxed the warm country bread into my bloodstream, and for a quarter on an hour I was happy.

While I'm one of those people who prefers a little break between the starter and the main course, provided that the waiters keep me topped up with bread, the gap on this occasion was painful. In the meantime, outside where we should have been sitting if it hadn't been for the wedding party, the speeches were in full flow, with the best man and his entourage sitting on a makeshift stage of bar stools set up in a row, the microphone journeying down the line in what looked like a question-and-answer session between the principals and the guests. What was surprising about the event was the lack of a bride.

The main course arrived eventually: *jambonette de lapin aux olives et son jus de cuisson*, which roughly translates as 'rabbit terrine in an olive-and-stock juice'. It was terrible. In effect, it was a rabbit terrine comatosed in the same tapenade that was on offer at the buffet counter, except that here it was sticky, over-salty and overbearing. At least it was served with a ration of the country bread, which made it somewhat palatable. As we dug in, the manager, a real-life Sybil Fawlty if ever there was one, told us in perfect English that the restaurant was closed the following evening – news to us – and asked us whether we wanted to skip dinner altogether or would we prefer to have dinner at lunchtime. Late as it was in the evening to be deciding these things, the thought of eating lunch in the corner of the restaurant at the discretion of the wedding party was a bridge too far for any market-gardener, let alone for two disgruntled tourists who had already had their bellyful of the local hospitality. We decided to skip dinner.

By the time we'd returned to the buffet counter for dessert, there were only leftovers, and of course the waiters had long since departed to the trenches for fear a guest might have the temerity to ask for an extra glass of wine or a jug of water – that is unless you were part of the wedding party, where somebody in that throng had obviously promised a king's ransom of a tip, and where service continued as usual. Not that that deterred me from scavenging through the leftovers, filling the plate with all sorts of creamed-up pastries and chocolate gob-fillers – much to my wife's embarrassment. Sensibly, she declined to partake in the wanton gluttony, and so, walking the journey of shame, I made my way back through the other guests, balancing my mountain of cakes – a tower of Babel to the altar of my greed – and drawing attention to myself and the Conscience like a leper ringing a bell.

Back at the table, the cakes were not as good as they looked – an appropriate ending to the dinner from hell – and I refused to eat them. However, my wife, embarrassed that I had taken the cakes in the first place, was now mortified that I hadn't at least made some effort to eat them. What was she worried about? It wasn't as if the food police were going to come barging in and grill us on why I'd had the temerity to take every last fancy to our table and then commit the cardinal sin of not eating them. *For Christ's sake,* I thought to myself, *it's getting worse: I'm married to a witch in charge of the food-police commission.* What was until then a pleasant bitch about the standards of French cooking in these parts soon descended into the classic 'eyes bigger than your belly' spiel, with my wife leading the case for the prosecution. So, to defend her honour, I forced myself on the chocolate log, which was over-sweet and obviously made with too much cocoa powder and not enough cocoa solids, and tucked into bits of the pastries, which, as usual in France, contain custard instead of cream. Yuck, yuck, yuck. If I've learned one thing over the last few months of trying to lose weight, it's not to eat something fatty you don't like just because it's there. If it's not up to scratch, leave it and move on to something better. If you're going to pig out on something that will add a centimetre to your waistline, be 100 percent sure that, pound for pound, this is the best lump of fat money can buy.

At a quarter past eleven, with my lower jaw dripping with the secondaries from a cream-and-chocolate bun fight, we left behind the remnants of a Provençal Mess and headed for our lofty perch, making our way through the wedding party's terraced paradise as the sound of café music struck up the accordions for '*J'y suis jamais allé*' – the theme tune from *Amélie* – while in a corner, laughing in unison, two twenty-something dolls serenaded a bloke in mock-uniform with what sounded like Edith Piaf's '*Mon Légionnaire*'.

The following morning, with the taste of the tapenade still painted to my tongue, we took a light French breakfast – coffee and a croissant – and, with the wailings of children and adults from the swimming pool echoing in our heads, headed out for the day. It was Sunday morning, and the sun was keen to put in a full shift. We decided to drive into Salon de Provence, about ten kilometres away down a winding road. Not having exercised for the last three days, I was beginning to feel edgy, and promised myself a swim that evening, when, with the hotel restaurant shut for the evening, there was sure to be no one around and I'd have the pool to myself.

Sunday lunch on holiday in France is one of my favourite meals, particularly if it's outside in the warm air: in the perfect ambience, it can be the laziest day of your life. We'd been to Salon before and knew the layout of the main streets. Having parked the car in what appeared to be the only road-side parking spot available, we went in search of Sunday lunch, skipping any thoughts of sightseeing.

We wanted something lively and outdoors, with good food to deflect the distraction of the previous night's fiasco. And as I hadn't eaten too much the previous night – notwithstanding the pig-out on the substandard cakes – and had had only a modicum of breakfast, I was hungry. We stopped at La Table d'Oscar, also called Pizzassimo, on rue de L'Horloge, where, on a smallish triangular-shaped thoroughfare over two levels, there were twenty-odd tables. Rue de L'Horloge runs down to Porte de

L'Horloge, a clock-towered arch which in the seventeenth century was the north gate to the town. For a time in the sixteenth century, Salon de Provence was home to Michel de Nostredame, or Nostra-damus, the French apothecary and soothsayer whose published prophecies many still claim predicted the rise of Napoleon and Hitler, Kennedy's assassination and, more recently, the flying of the planes into the World Trade Center. Nostradamus's old house was around the corner from where we were seated. So, essentially, we were in Nostradamus's manor: the up-and-down side streets where the great seer sought inspiration for his forecasts on his way past the local Franciscan chapel, St Michel – which apparently he didn't fancy as a place of worship, and which to this day doesn't appear to do much business. You like to think that the Big N had once told the Church 'I told you so'. Anyway, every so often a crowd of sightseers knapsacked past with their designer sunglasses and multi-lens cameras capturing scenes the wise old chancer could never have predicted.

Sitting comfortably with a good view of everything around us, we wondered if Nostradamus – the Michel Roux of his day, particularly when his *Treatise on Cosmetics and Conserves* was published – was expecting us. Or if he ever imagined that the restaurant, now serving Sunday lunch, would share its forecourt with an old garage across from it, spreading its tables right up to the garage door, or whether a dumpy middle-aged man would walk in among us and make for the public phone-box to the side and begin what turned out to be a twenty-five-minute animated phone-call while the patrons sat and absorbed what seems to come naturally in these parts.

Ever since Saumur on the first day of our holiday, I had tried to eat sensibly, so much so that I hadn't put on any weight, and in my everyday clothes – T-shirt, shorts and sandals – I was for the most part comfortable, with all the wobbly bits having room to manoeuvre. A lot of this was down to not asking for *pommes frites* with everything from pizza to steak, although I craved them; at the Conscience's insistence, I instead had local country salads, which usually heave with smoked-duck breasts, foie gras, lardons, gizzards and a few puy lentils or haricot beans over a mountain of green leaves, hiding a vinaigrette dressing below. To my belly, eyes and consciousness, it's a salad for a king.

Having ordered the wine, a delicate local rosé, I sat back on my throne, the psychological reflexes in my head freewheeling down to my gut with messages of intent. Like Pavlov, who up until the death of his son – fighting on the wrong side in the aftermath of the Russian Revolution – was a bit manic about when and how he ate his lunch, I have a similar Pavlovian desire to eat breakfast in the morning, lunch in the middle of the day and dinner in the evening, three square meals that carry me through the day. The problem has always been that I could never replicate this at home, where I'm unable, for the most part, to marshal myself away from the ruinous snacks. On holidays in the company of the Conscience, I rarely stray from the path. In fact, I've often thought of organising specialist holidays for fat blokes where, for a month in the year, you plonk them in Aix or Salon de Provence, with their ball-and-chains, and let nature do the rest.

The meal arrives. *Salade aux quatre fromages* for the wife and *salade gourmande* 'for the *mano*', says the waiter, eager to show off his English. I don't correct him, say thanks and good luck, and before he has turned his back, the sprinters' starting gun goes off in my head, and I'm relishing the delights of the local cuisine. A look from the wife cautions me to slow down, and I do, munching the salad leaves and livers in an open sandwich. I try desperately to disprove the myth that *salade gourmande* is a salad for a greedy person, and for most part I succeed, enjoying the luxury of a fatty salad untainted by chips. A couple of lemon-sorbet *Colonel*s later, we walk around the town, which is obviously in hibernation – it's definitely Sunday – stopping to sit on a local bench, as usual stuffed to the gills, to the detriment of my life, like you'd force-feed a goose to make foie gras.

We ended up at the zoo – Zoo de la Barben – about five minutes' drive from Salon. What were we to do for the afternoon in Salon? I'd had a drink or two over a two-hour lunch, and there weren't too many attractions within walking or short-driving distance that we hadn't already been to – mindful that we didn't want to push it with *les flics*. The thought of going back to an empty closed-for-dinner hotel-restaurant called Fawlty Domaine, with obviously no food for later, was not exactly appetising. As you can see, I was already thinking about the next meal.

So, Zoo de la Barben it was, a thirty-three-hectare zoo on the road between Pelissanne and St Cannat. It was the middle of the day and, by God, it was warm. The type of day you just know you'll need liquids, and plenty of them. By this stage, we were feeling lazy and not really sure how much of the zoo we wanted to see. We knew that, while the zoo authorities said that you could fly around it in a minimum of two hours, you really should take four hours, and we were happy that the facility was closing in less than three hours.

Having paid our admission, the first obstacle we encountered was gravity. The zoo was built on a high hill that overlooks the valley and the surrounding countryside. While I was conscious that I could do with some exercise, the thought of pulling myself and my wife – who at this stage was tiring – up a steep gradient wasn't a training schedule that could possibly have my name on it. Luckily, and before one of us had a heart attack just thinking about how Chris Bonington would have risen to the summit with one hand carrying his Bovril, Le Petit Train – one of those touristy miniature trains that seem to be everywhere nowadays – whistled along and gave us a ride to the top for a shiny new euro each.

From atop the plateau, we squinted out over the zoo, which spread out across the hillside. It wasn't particularly busy: mostly youngish families out for a Sunday afternoon. In fact, there wasn't anyone in the zoo in their late fifties, although I didn't check the age of any of the animals. All the blokes seemed to be on a concentration-camp diet, with scrawny, wiry bodies that celebrated neck muscles and ribcages. They also weren't aware of the rest-day custom of wearing a shirt or T-shirt, and nearly every male went bare-chested. There was a mania for body art and tattoos, with all kinds of serpents, crocodiles and penguins pushing for arm space between daggers, swords, French emblems and flags. Sadly, there were also a couple of what looked like Ma Mère et Mon Père, although, such is the nature of tattoos, that it's not really the sort of thing you can inspect casually without provoking an unwelcome response. The tattoos were not confined to the men. Several of the women had them, and again in all shapes and sizes. And then there was me, with no tattoo anywhere, although with a pen I could have joined the dots on my white skin, between my mosquito bites, bloodstains and bruising, and signalled to the world around both my ankles and my left arm *Vive La France*. As for the thought of discarding my shirt: no chance, and to hell with being in the middle of nature.

After topping up on water and a bottle of orange that was not cold enough to either hydrate or satisfy, we made our way around the zoo at a snail's pace, staying in the shade as much as we could, and taking photographs of the animals, like every other tourist. What was exceptional about this particular zoo was the lack of space given to some of the animals, who were expected to perform, day in, day out, cramped into corners and side-stages like inhabitants in a Lego village. As you'd expect, Orwell's prognosis was alive and flying the flag in the heart of Provence: 'All animals are equal, but some animals are more equal than others.' This was never better illustrated than in the Siberian tiger enclosure, where three Esso pin-ups – who were all, at least, entitled to an Animal Hero, Second Class, and if I caught sight of Monsieur Jones I'd have told him so – were bound within the perimeter of a cage that you'd fit into your town-house back garden. There they were, these huge hunks of cat-flesh, whose natural inclination is to hunt, trap and mug deer, wild pigs and water buffalo, while doing the training routine of a decathlon athlete, stuck in a confinement where they had to be inventive to stay active. By the time we'd got there, I, along with the animals, was considering dinner, and the tigers were on patrol pacing their countdown to the wishful thinking of ripped antelope *à la provençal*.

Staring as I was, the fat Irishman, through bulletproof glass at these youngish-looking lean tigers, taking snaps to show the folks back home, it struck me how obviously stupid I was, my nose glued to the glass cage, watching animals exercising. Meanwhile, on the other side of the enclosure, the caged felines methodically walked along a thin, twenty-foot promenade – what I presume you'd call a catwalk – 153 times before I could get the bloody camera to work and in such a way as to get the cats in focus and in a good light. Finally, just on cue, the first cat in line stared straight into my eyes as I took the snap, no doubt recognising in my face either dinner or the resemblance of something big enough to eat. Watching the cats, who had not for one moment broken stride, I realised that even the dumb animal looking at the fat git through the glass knew that he had to exercise. Five photos later, one of the cats had made his way down to a water feature – apparently, tigers and jaguars are the Olympic swimmers of the big-cat population, although obviously they don't carry whiskey with them to the toilet – by the side fence, where he walked backwards and forwards over a ten-foot narrow stretch again and again. It was enough to make an acrobat dizzy, and proof, if proof was needed, that too much exercise is bad for you.

By that stage, we'd had enough, and I was getting a bit peckish dreaming about what I was going to have for dinner. Worn out and over-exercised, we made our way back to the hotel, stopping off in Salon for a pizza, bread and a little cheese. When we got to the hotel, we were amazed to see an elongated railway-crossing-style gate blocking the main avenue to the hotel entrance. There was no way in and no way out. Getting out of the car and scratching our heads – cartoon characters lost in someone else's storyline – we recognised an intercom system of sorts sticking up out of the ground, a lone sentinel (something you'd have expected Neil Armstrong to stick in the ground if this were the first great hiccup for mankind) guarding the gate. Locating what looked like a microphone with a key-pad, we pressed the button nearest the microphone a couple of times, the alien in us looking at our fingers, eyeing the button and then pressing it almost in slow motion, hoping for a response, and then a little more aggressively, conscious that the pizza, propped up like a hostage in the back seat of the car, was getting cold. We were polite at first, and used a touch of the happy-go-lucky vernacular – '*Bonsoir, bonsoir. S'il vous plaît, ouvrez la porte*'. Politeness didn't work. Then it got a little more serious, the pizza burning a hole in my mind: 'Open the bleeding gate, you bastards.' All to no avail, and it was already 7.30 PM.

We then had a penguin moment, looking at ourselves like Mr and Mrs Emperor, who've just arrived home to find John and Oko wearing their bathrobes: what do we do next, Aptenodytes Forsteri? We tried a bit more charm, dragging up from the depths of our memories any phrase that might get the attention of someone in the hotel. The time was really running out for the pizza, so much so that – incredibly for a man in my condition – I was going off it. We rang the hotel's phone number, repeatedly, but to no avail. If there was a receptionist at home or on duty, she was cleaning the floor of the swimming pool, underwater.

We thought about jumping over the gate, running up the hundred-yard-long avenue and inflicting blue murder on anyone officious we could get our hands on. All the time, the hostage in the back seat got colder, while the blood in my veins congealed with anger. Rage and hunger are a bad cocktail in my body-works, and usually in these situations the jackboots in my head march towards the end zone, where the kettle of a humanitarian catastrophe is ready to boil over. It's Baader Meinhof territory. And the pizza had better watch out, because I was liable to pull the hood off its head, march it on to waste land, and do what Andreas Baader might have done: shot it straight in the forehead between the mozzarella and the oregano.

However, the touch-tone key-pad below the microphone offered us further distraction, and a chance to 'Pink Panther' the key-code. Obviously it had a key-code. Why not check the key? Wouldn't that be a good place to mark a key-code for your guests? The key was certainly big enough: it resembled something that you'd imagine the Count of Monte Cristo was locked up with. *Where's the key?* Found it. *For your starter for ten, pretty wife, does the word 'key-code' appear on our rock of a key?* Yes. *Bingo. So what is it?* Someone's rubbed it out. *What do you mean, someone's rubbed it out? You're joking, aren't you?* No. *Show me the bleeding key.* And sure enough, where someone had decoratively written in fancy calligraphy the word 'key-code', obviously followed by the code, someone else from *The Shawshank Redemption* had taken a rock-hammer to what was once a five- or possibly six-digit cipher.

I made a beeline for the pizza, with the strong intention of tying it to the gate with a note: *Pizza pour O'Doherty, pour qui ces ignobles entraves, ces fers dès longtemps préparés?* ('for whom these vile shackles, these long-prepared irons?' – a verse of 'La Marseillaise'). My wife, who is usually the first to crack in these sort of situations, was already showing the early symptoms of the equivalent of Stockholm syndrome – where the hostage-taker shows loyalty to the hostage – and intervened and calmed me down, telling me that surely this wasn't the sort of obstacle to come between me and my dinner. And of course she was right, but it was appeasement, and certainly not the sort of action that was going to get us in the gate. No, this called for violence.

A rational moment later, we were back to square one, staring at the keypad for inspiration. It came in a thunderbolt from a parley between my tastebuds and whatever rationality I had left. Thinking out loud, I thought that most people never change their alarm codes, computer gates or child locks after they are installed. Thus '1-2-3-4' is the most commonly used alarm code in the world – if you remove the millions of Chinese not familiar with the Arabic method – and was worth trying. *So, in our survey of one million hotels around the world, what was the most common key-code used on gates to keep the guests out of their bedrooms? You said: '1-2-3-4'. Our survey said: '1-2-3-4'.* Bingo. Without a second's hesitation, the gate calmly retracted and slid back into the open-sesame position. This was all a bit of shock, because I was sure that in my hurry I hadn't pressed the four. Nevertheless it had worked, and we ran back to the jalopy, started it up, and drove up the main avenue, as the gate closed slowly behind us. We then turned right and parked her under the trees outside the hotel reception.

The hotel was as peaceful as the first day in the Garden of Eden, or the aftermath of a Quatermass experiment. We got out of the car and stared around, looking for any visible sign of life. Not a sound. I took the pizza out of the back seat, along with other bits and pieces, and piled them in my arms pyramid-style. We made our way into the hotel lobby, where nothing moved except, spookily, the office computer against the wall, which was humming that noise that tells you it's not a fridge. We raised our voices slightly to make ourselves heard: *'Bonsoir, bonsoir.'*

Nothing. We decided to make our way over to the restaurant. Again, nothing. It was quiet and deserted. They were right when they said that the restaurant would be closed on the Sunday evening. It was eight o'clock, and still somewhere in the high twenties centigrade, and we were now getting thirsty as well as very hungry. A couple of jugs of cold refreshing water wouldn't go amiss, and you could throw in a dozen ice cubes while you were at it. So where do you find the ice in someone else's hotel, where there are no windows, in the dark? We went in and around the shadowy restaurant, looking for any sign of life, or at least the direction to the fridge. Again we made ourselves known: 'Bonsoir, bonsoir.' Still nothing. We went back outside, thinking we'd find somebody before we took matters into our own hands. While I walked around the outhouses in the courtyard, my wife went up a stone staircase to what looked like living accommodation, but could easily pass as a stone stairway to a parapet. By the time she reached the top step, she heard voices coming from a room just inside a rather spooky door. She went inside and saw, by the light from a computer screen, two blokes sitting in their underpants mesmerised by the computer in front of them. Not wanting to disturb whatever pastime they were up to, she asked them politely did they know was there anybody about from the hotel, and where could she get some cold water and ice. Both answers came back in the negative, and she returned to me as quickly as possible, not wanting to oversee their business for any longer than was needed.

In the courtyard I was now on hunger death row, and of a mind to leave immediately, chucking the pizza into the fountain in the middle of the circular restaurant. I was beginning to soothe the food like a father rocking a baby to sleep, going out of my mind with hunger. Would it be a good idea to pack up and leave in search of a hotel for the night? It would be like the holy family and the baby pizza looking for accommodation. And then there was the problem of paying for our stay: how would we manage that? We would obviously have to return, to explain the situation, no matter what happened. No, thanks. Besides, could we even get out at all? What if the code I'd entered was a lucky one-off, and wouldn't work a second time? I was fucked if I was going to go up and ask the local Ant and Dec (or should that be 'Ant and Underpant') for the key to the way out.

Just then, an elderly couple approached us, obviously tourists, also staying at the hotel: they didn't look the type who burgled hotels on a Sunday. She was one of those quaint little women you'd expect to find gossiping in *Emmerdale* or doing all the work for the *Midsomer Murder* fair. She was English to the core and brought up believing that everything was really nice. Once we got talking, she laughed at everything we said with a chuckle and a shrug, adding, on the subject of the French: 'It's your foreigner, isn't it?' He was originally from Llanelli and straight out of the Welsh Guards, a soldier in his youth who had never made it past private, but a proud individual nevertheless who had one of those accents from *Zulu* and finished every sentence with 'you see'. *Now retired, you see. Drove down from Cheshire on Wednesday, you see. Spent a weekend in the south of England, headed for France, you see.*

While she just laughed, he, a tipple or two in love with life, stuck out his chest through the whitest, most ironed shirt I have ever seen, and told us the rest of their holiday story. She continued to chuckle, correcting him when needed and reassuring us that he was being economical with the truth. 'A pizza, I see,' he said, recognising the international takeaway box that was now only lukewarm in my arms – but still warm enough for me not to chuck it away. Would they like to join us for a bite, I asked – hoping that I wouldn't have to share. 'No,' says he, 'only had a bite earlier, you see. Not hungry, you see. You go on. Eat away, boyo.'

The conversation turned quickly to the deserted Hostellerie du Domaine de la Reynaude, which we now knew housed a magnificent half-dozen – Ant and Underpant, the Welsh Wizard and Mrs England, the Conscience and me. Did the retired couple find anything strange about the hotel and the people who worked there, and the fact that at half eight on a Sunday evening there wasn't a sinner for miles who could assist you if you had a heart attack, give you a glass of cold water or at least offer you a clean pair of underpants while you waited for an ambulance.

We told them about the gate. 'What?' says the Welsh Guard. 'Closed, you say? I don't believe it. You have a code, you say? Might work. 1-2-3-4?' you say. 'I'm going to try it. If not, I'm going to climb over the bloody gate and escape. No one stops me going for a bloody Sunday-evening walk. Who do they think they are? Zulus?'

And so we departed, the Welsh Wizard gagging for a challenge on his holidays, his poor wife behind him, giggling and yet seriously worried that her husband would do himself a injury. We went straight to our room, opened a bottle of moderately cold champagne and cut up the cold pizza. A slice and a half of pizza later, and having only nibbled on the other goodies, we had had enough. The weather was too warm, the food was too cold, and it tasted like dried cardboard coated with cheap tomato paste and rubbery cheese. Disappointed in the extreme, I started to read; within an hour, I was asleep.

The following day, we had breakfast – which, after the previous night's shenanigans, wasn't enough, as usual – and toyed with the idea of saying goodbye to the circus. It was Monday morning, and we could easily take to the road and find somewhere where the service couldn't be worse. However, with the heat, the humidity and a long holiday, we were tired from travelling, and a little lazy. We didn't feel up to driving around looking for accommodation, two days into our three-day stay. So we decided to stay. We did search out Madame Fawlty and pointed out our grievances to her about the previous night.

Her reaction? 'So?'

'So what are you going to do about it, madame?'

'You got in OK?'

'Eventually. We didn't know we needed a code. No one told us. You didn't tell us we needed a code.'

'It's on your keyring.'

'No, it isn't. Look, someone with a rock-hammer chiselled it off.'

'So?'

'So what are you going to do about it?'

'So you were waiting to get in, and you got in. So?'

'We wanted water and some ice.'

At this, she ran into the kitchen and came back with ice and a bottle of water. 'No charge,' says she. 'Happy?'

Well, not really, but that was as far as we were going to get with it. We forgot to ask what we would do in an emergency or if we had to go out after hours to see Provence, because we were supposed to be tourists, and tourists go out, don't they – although apparently not from this hotel.

That evening at dinner in the restaurant, we were seated outside, at the entrance to the inner dining area. We were facing two English couples whose voices squeaked like hinges that hadn't been oiled since the Coronation. Ten feet away, sipping our aperitifs, we could hear their conversation ominously swing a garden gate open, as if Dracula or the ghost of Tutankhamen was expected. Sadly, the only ghoulish offering was the sight of *pommes frites* being served in a French restaurant to one of the men – which, from a gourmand's perspective, was probably as frightening as if Peter Cushing, Christopher Lee and the rest of the Hammer House cast appeared in your bedroom at 4 o'clock in the morning. From my perspective, suffering moderately from lack of fast food, and definitely in chip remission – I hadn't had chips for nearly a month – this was like offering drugs or alcohol to everybody except the reformed addict.

And I wasn't the only one who was put out. The Englishman's friend didn't receive any chips, but did get lashings of *pommes de terre*. For a moment, the man stared at the potatoes – which had been washed to their pale-yellow skins, boiled and then served in probably unsalted butter – before darting a glance at the oil-soaked chips, which looked crispy and enticing. His hair was the most noticeable thing about him: it was unwashed, as though he'd just discovered grunge, and was waiting for it to grow. He also wore the type of green-check shirt that gardeners wear in winter, although from what we could hear him saying – he didn't recognise any of the vegetables on his plate – it occurred to me that he had never grown vegetables or flowers in his life. He offered some polite comment to his circle on the noticeable lack of chips on his plate compared to that of his compatriot, and started to eat. The others ignored him, or didn't hear him, while, further inside the restaurant, I could hear Mrs England from the previous night describe to her company in a soft tone: 'It's your foreigner, isn't it?' The Englishman in front of me didn't hear her, but continued to stare at his companion's plate with envy, too shy to say that he had been severely wronged, and that no amount of yellow-skinned buttered potatoes was going to make up for it. Oddly, his wife, who was sitting beside him, had her back turned to him, as if side-saddling a horse for the hunt. For the rest of the meal, the conversation squeaked irritatingly this way and that. While I wished that I didn't have a can of WD40, the man sitting opposite his friend with the unwashed hair picked at his food with his fingers like a king, while his wife ate with the grace of a queen.

Behind us, a baby – no more than a year or a year and a half old – was put into her walker and left to her own devices in the restaurant's courtyard. She quickly made her way to a water fountain in the middle of the outdoor terrace, which was home to two particularly noisy frogs. Seeing the fountain as a bit of a challenge, she circumnavigated it twenty-five times – we know it was twenty-five times, because Mother England was counting – her legs turning the walker with a speed and generosity that is rarely mentioned in those safety adverts that tell you that baby-walkers aren't the safest form of toddler exercise or that the International Olympic Committee has outlawed such training aids.

Anyway, luckily no one attacked the child with a bamboo or any other impediment, although I'm sure that there were one or two spies from various European and American Olympic committees checking out whether she was qualified, through the granny rule, to represent their countries. On pure athletic merit, you could see what Marion Jones or any of those other American wonder kids look like before they end up hiring Johnnie Cochran types when they fail a drugs test before their sixteenth birthdays. If this child had been born in the former GDR, she would already be in training for the 2020 Olympics and the gruel in her baby's bottle would be laced with EPO and every other growth hormone you could think of. What event was the child to grace? Well, by the way she flung her rattle out of the walker and poleaxed the poor frog, whose voice croaked with the innocence of an aggrieved operatic bystander, the child's future could very well be in the javelin or discus.

During all this time, the service at our table continued to worsen. The starter, at the buffet, was miserly as usual, and gone by the time we arrived. When we pointed this out, the waiter looked at us in shock but said nothing, playing the old 'We're not sure what you're saying in your pidgin French' routine. Our wine was nearly frozen again when it arrived, the fruit hiding in its overcoat somewhere in the skin of the bottle, and the coup de grâce, the main course – *poêlé de légumes à l'estragon*, or pot-roasted vegetables, with enough tarragon to cure a dentist's surgery of toothache or a reptile village of rattlesnake bites – arrived even colder. Knowing full well that the cold dinners were a button-push away from being blitzed in the microwave, I picked at some of the potatoes which accompanied the dish – my wife content to leave everything as it was – and called over the waiter, when I could find one, to explain that our main courses were cold.

This is where obesity and food greed is at its worst. You want to make a point that the food is cold and inedible, but not before eating a few of the sides bits, hoping you might get more. Stroppy to the point of nearly swiping the tablecloth off the table, the waiter marched away with the plates. Another waiter returned after about three minutes – my plate obviously missing the potatoes I'd eaten – and us our plates, careful not to give me the plate with my wife's piping-hot potatoes. It was blatant: we know you ate the potatoes, and we know you know we're going to just heat them up in the microwave, and really we don't give a toss, so do your worst. It was like a slap in the face, or having a big muck-filled chevalier's gauntlet dropped into your soup.

I was too hungry to complain, although if I'd had better French I'm sure I could have at least explained to the police later why I had assaulted the waiter with the dinner, if it had come to that, or at least pointed out that, no, I didn't want the microwave touching my dinner and would they kindly take away the re-heats and serve me up a new dish especially prepared. But by the time this had occurred to me, I had nearly finished my meal and – to my wife's annoyance – was asking for more bread, to sweep up the overbearingly pungent sauce. When we got to the dessert counter for the finale, what was left resembled a bun fight among the Spindrift crew in *The Land of the Giants*.

Back at our table, a waitress brought us a glass of champagne each: a peace offering, you could call it, to mitigate for any one of half a dozen mishaps. However, the speed with which she muttered the apology had us wondering if they were on the house or an order misdirected to our table. With her discourteous growl, her lack of eye-contact, and the fact that we got the feeling she would have preferred to throw the drinks over us, we concluded that the young woman would never make it in public relations, politics or diplomacy. A person who is incapable of delivering a pizza should not be sent to deliver an apology. For the record, the champagne was drinkable.

The following morning, after all sorts of shenanigans over the bill (Had we paid a deposit? To whom had we sent it? No, we didn't receive it. How much was it again?), which took nearly an hour to sort out, we eventually left the Domaine for good at around eleven o'clock. Taking to the road is something I've always loved, especially the uncertainty as to where we might end up, and that particular day was no different. It was the Tuesday before the Friday-evening departure from Roscoff for Cork. We decided that we'd had enough of Provence on this holiday and that it was time to head a little closer to the ferry. So far on the holiday, I had done little to lose weight, although I was sure that the extra salads, and plenty of water, had loosened a notch on my shorts, as opposed to loosening the stitching.

On the road again, we drove towards the Rhône Valley – specifically, Vacqueyras. In the past, we had occasionally stayed in a pretty nineteenth-century house-cum-hotel, the Hôtel Montmirail, a hideaway close to the wine region of Gigondas and just outside the village of Vacqueyras, in the instep at the foot of the Dentelles mountains. It is surrounded by vineyards, olive trees and peace, and is the sort of place where no one makes noise above the turning of the next page in a book. While the rooms are a little tight on personality and space, and with poor views if you get a room at the back, the food and wine are superb, the hospitality is first class, and there is a heated swimming pool.

The journey up the A7 from Salon past Avignon towards Orange didn't take long once we'd bypassed the traffic around Salon. We drove through those little villages that make up the first and second tiers of Rhône viticulture. By this time, I was Pavlov's excited greyhound, dreaming as I licked my lips about lunch. I've often thought that this is where I could eat sensibly for the rest of my life. With such heat and sunshine – the temperature settles in the mid-thirties, if not higher, in summer – I'd certainly eat less (fast food is a much more complicated option) and, having to drink water regularly, I'm sure that my lifestyle would be a lot healthier.

We have lunch at one of our favourite restaurants, L'Oustalet in Gigondas. Having had a pithy breakfast at the Domaine and spent so much valuable eating time arguing over the bill, I'm running close to the black needle of emptiness, and lunch can't come fast enough. L'Oustalet is in the shade of the trees, the view reaching around the *place* and out over the valley below. In all the years we've been coming to Gigondas, we have never witnessed rain, and the sun is always on its best behaviour. In a region where the wine has such a reputation, we have never seen rainfall. And we've never witnessed the Mistral either, come to think of it – that angry Rhône swirl of a rocket whose presence is as fierce as its reputation.

We are embedded with the locals, and away from an American family, who, as usual, are asking those next to them what they do for a living. Across from where we sit, a group of middle-aged men arrive in the *place* on bikes, panting and gasping for air. They are dressed in racing shorts and shirts, although none of them have helmets or appear to be carrying water. Grey- or white-haired, and nearly all in their late fifties or early sixties, they walk around in search of a water carrier or tap, bow-legged and obviously saddle-sore from their exertions. Finally, they congregate around two Swiss-registered micro-buses. The two drivers are similar in age to the cyclists, although with heavier and rounder faces and stomachs. As I tuck into my first piece of real bread of the day, I hear the Americans in the restaurant behind me complaining: 'My God, no one here speaks American.' They are too stupid or too ignorant to recognise the odd English or Irish person in their midst, playing a blinder with their French. Two thoughts come to me. First, what is it with men spending all their life exercising with other men? And second, by the time I'm their age, will I be driving the bus or panting and puffing the bike up the hill?

It has always seemed a little odd to me that men have a fascination with doing physical pursuits with other men, whether it's Gaelic, soccer, rugby or, in this case, cycling. Right from the time we're born, we're more likely to join other men in physical exercise, instead of investing more time in other games, like the mixed-doubles tennis team, where access to women is far greater. Why is it that the majority of men prefer to keep their games and women separate?

Cycling around France has always been on my to-do list, specifically following the route of the Tour de France. Obviously, at this weight, it's always going to be difficult, and would probably take me six months. Alpe d'Huez, the legendary mountaintop finish, holds a particular fascination. Probably on the top table of famous Tour finishes, the climb is 13.8 kilometres, at an average gradient of more than 8 percent, and includes twenty-one hairpin turns, which twist the most willing participant into submission. Not the sort of exercise any bloke in the 17- or 18-stone division should attempt. But then again, if I was properly fit, this is the type of exercise I'd love to do every day of my life, which – and I can't be sure about this without doing a vox pop – isn't the type of comment you'd expect to get from a person with my weight problems. Maybe I'm destined always to be a greedy bastard who can't be trusted with a knife and fork, but hey, if I could only convert some of my enthusiasm into real physical endeavour, I might at least be able to reach some sort of accommodation that balances over-eating with over-exercise. It's not ideal, but it is one solution. Anyway, the Italian rider Marco Pantani, who was found dead on St Valentine's Day 2004 in a hotel room in Rimini from cocaine poisoning, still holds the record for the climb, at 36 minutes 50 seconds, which he achieved in 1995. In my present condition, it would probably take me thirty-six hours to complete, and I'd need to be met by a fleet of ambulances to take every one of my organs individually to hospital, because each part of my body would fall off with the exhaustion. And like the two blokes driving the buses, I'd be in no condition to throw my leg over a saddle again. Not that I can see much satisfaction in driving a dumpy brand new bus while my mates are having all the fun.

Two days later, we were back home. Despite the temptations, promises and hopes, my weight was the same as when we'd left, thirty days previously.

JULY

PROGRESS

AUGUST

HEALTH, LIVER, BACK AND BUM

I have had hole trouble for a couple of years. Hole trouble? It happens like this. One minute you're running around pulling weeds by the hair on their heads, scoffing a sly snack box somewhere in suburbia or even holding the ladder as the wife is washing the windows, when suddenly, without prior sensation, you have all the paraphernalia of the bum's rush and the early-warning signs of a major evacuation. Throwing secateurs, breaded chicken and scaffolding behind you, you drag your bones to any available toilet, whether it's down stairs, up escalators or behind someone's shed. Assuming the position, you press those buttons in the mind that open the release chutes. The command signal goes down the line from commander to marine gunner, and once everything seems in tip-top shape, you readjust your position for maximum comfort and shout 'Fire!' And then you wait. And wait. You give the order again: 'Fire!' Again, nothing happens. Realising it's all been a bit of a false alarm, you pick up the jocks, trousers, shorts, swimming togs, whatever you're wearing, tie everything in place and wash your hands.

No sooner are you walking away than the bum's rush comes again, this time much more ferociously. You drop everything again, post-haste, even faster than the last time, and dive bum-first on to the spot of fresh ground or toilet bowl. This time, the gunner doesn't wait for your command, and fires automatically. Fire. Fire. Fire. But again nothing happens. Frustration kicks in and the inevitable bellyache joins the parade, so you rub your stomach like crazy, hoping to alleviate some of the discomfort around the wide expanses of Bellyland. You stand up. You sit down. You do a few star jumps. You even jog on the spot. A loud knock comes to the door, if there is one. 'I'll be out in a minute!' you scream back, in one of those angry verbals. Suddenly, faced with company, and the thoughts of a queue, the ability to 'go' vanishes. However, you dare not move. Something is definitely coming; it's just that you don't know when. You pray for deliverance. The knock comes on the door again. 'I told you, I'll be out in a minute!' you scream back, the anxiety doing overtime.

You prepare a family pack of toilet paper, convinced that this is going to be the diaspora to end all diasporas, and that there are bound to be casualties. You push a little harder and feel the strain on your temples as if you're going to burst a blood vessel. It's hard to believe, crouched in such as way that your bum is a foot and a half from the ground, but you feel the pull of gravity and the sensation of vertigo. If you weren't artificially sitting down, you feel that you could easily fall down. You steady yourself. You make that grunt of desperation that follows constipation around like a horrible twin. You may as well be waiting for Godot in a toilet, or ten thousand Godots, wondering did Beckett write any or all of it sitting on a toilet, constipated. You realise how Vladimir must have felt waiting, waiting, waiting, believing that yes, he'll definitely come – the toilet, a metaphysical tree. You wonder would any of those avant-garde playwrights ever consider setting Beckett's play in a toilet with Vladimir, his jocks around his ankles, sitting on the bowl, and Estragon asking inquisitively: 'You're sure it was here? That we were to meet?' You feel as if you're an inmate of a prison – it could be Lüttringhausen or San Quentin – and you're waiting, waiting, waiting for release.

It's eleven Dunkirks in half the space, and the Germans are sending an extra fourteen divisions, most of which are outside banging on the bloody door. 'I'll be out in a minute!' you shout for the last time, as euphoria finally comes slowly down the track. Yes, yes, yes. Thank you, God, thank you, you cry, thumping the wall with your fist, milking the goodness of creation and the satisfaction of a job well done. It's a little sore, achingly sore, but no sooner has the visitor arrived than he's gone.

Clean-up completed, you note a touch of blood in your stool. Specks, really, but blood-red. Tomato skins, even, although it dawns on you that you haven't had anything off a vine for weeks. You look a little closer: red, definitely, but maybe not enough to worry anyone. So you leave it, flush it away – metaphorically as well. Gone. That is, until the next time. No matter how confident I am that I've flushed the bejaysus away, the worm of scepticism rattles the cage of my self-assurance.

I've always been a sceptic, whatever the circumstances. Even that time when I interviewed the psychic. I didn't give her a chance, realising that it was baloney from the start. I remember the way I'd spent the whole weekend planning my week, with as much military precision as Rommel's pursuit across the Tagliamento, when the phone rings. It's an emissary from the extrasensory practitioner, apologising that the morning interviews have over-shot and would the freelance bloke from the *Irish Times* mind coming in a little early because the psychic has forgotten that she needs to catch an early-evening train back to Belfast. Thus the interview will be shorter than I'd hoped. I'm not impressed. I've eaten fortune cookies that were more predictable. But hey, I'm interested, sceptically interested. I agree.

And so I hurry through mid-afternoon traffic, dodging every other nomad who has an early appointment or who's trying to avoid drive-time headaches, passing pedestrians with death wishes side-armed with cots and baby-pushing machines, preparing my questions as I go. Was she expecting to overrun with the other interviews? Did she know I'd be wearing a green mac? Does she know if the Arnotts car park is full? Should I try the Jervis Street Shopping Centre? Will I get clamped if I park on Abbey Street? And more importantly, will the long-haired brother in the chartreuse microbus ahead of me ever make up his mind if he's turning right or left?

I arrive for the interview. The venue is closed during the day and they're saving on electricity. It's dark, really dark. I'm ushered in as if I'm the last electrician in Europe, and am intro-duced to the psychic and her manager. Psychics apparently need managers.

We begin. Firstly, she doesn't do futures. Not to worry, my car is safe in the Arnotts car park anyway. Secondly, she doesn't give private readings during interviews to penny-pinching journalists. And thirdly, I get the sales pitch. The success at Edinburgh (questionable), the new Irish and British tour, and the format for the show: woman stands on stage and connects dead person with living relative in audience. Easy work if you can get it.

So tell us, what's a clairvoyant? 'Well, I prefer to be called a psychic – someone who communicates information from loved ones who have passed over to the other side. I have been able to do this since I was five years old, when I would wake up in the middle of the night very frightened, having heard voices. I didn't know what was happening. I thought everybody heard these people. I didn't understand it was only me. In the beginning I was sceptical.

'Even in England, where I studied courses in business studies, sociology and psychology, I was still sceptical and would only do my party tricks for fun. My family were also sceptical about what was happening but were convinced when I saw my grandmother after she died. She died when I was fourteen. I have been blind since birth. I have no visual perception of colours, yet I was able to tell my family what my grandmother wore in detail. I was able to describe colours I've never seen. It convinced them and me that something unusual had happened.'

So how do you communicate with the dead? 'Well, I have a team on the other side who talk to me.' My ears prick up. A team? An invisible team? Now we're getting somewhere. Like a football team? Not quite. 'I have eight members on my team on the other side,' she says, as nonchalantly as any heart specialist would roll-call his portfolio of juniors. 'Eight members?' I think out loud. I ask, Billy Connolly-like: 'And who might they be?' 'There's Patrick, Gerard [a former psychiatric nurse from Cork who only died a few years ago – I bet he's run off his feet], James, John, Brendan and two Egyptian seers from 2000 BC, called Guiveraugh and Haran-Tut-Ra', whom she calls Tut, but I'm not to mistake him for Tutankhamen. Don't worry, I won't. I have done my Egyptology one-times-tables and I know that the boy pharaoh ruled Egypt from 1333 until 1323 BC, so I know that your sun-worshipping soothsayers have never heard of him, unless they watch the History Channel. She apologises for her spellings (of the Egyptian guys' names); she has never been asked to spell them before. I forget to ask her who the eighth member of the team is, and why there's a gender bias, and how come she has two Egyptians working for her in the first place. But hey, this is a multicultural society, and maybe the other side is no different. Except, of course, working on the other side, you don't need a work permit, and if she ever lays them off, they won't have to wait two years for social-welfare payments.

So tell us, what does this little Hiberno-Egyptian entourage do? Besides being offspring from a very fertile imagination. Don't tell me. They work for Keyser Söze? No? OK, are they a team of creative writers? No? Do they prefer Roddy Doyle to James Joyce? OK, I give up, what do they do? Wait for it. 'They all have their own jobs. Some work in communications. Some in security, making sure everything is OK and warning me of danger. Some work in teaching, and one is in public relations, preparing me for interviews.' I half-expect her to tell me that the eighth person is Bunny or Terry something, but I don't go there. Also, I'd like to have a few quiet words with the person advising her on time-management – a candidate for the sack, if ever there was one.

So how do you manage to keep a conversation going with eight people? 'Easy – they're on shift work.' Shift work? I can hear characters from Monty Python sketches telling me from Grail-like towers: 'She's *making it up*.' I wonder if Spike Milligan ever did Egyptian impressions. If not, he must be having a right old giggle on the other side listening to this.

On a roll, I delve a little deeper. Has she ever been the victim of an ET abduction? (I have read that some clairvoyants have been abducted.) 'It's possible,' she says, but doesn't think so. The seriousness of her answer reminds me that this is a vulnerable woman who for whatever reason strongly believes she has a gift and is prepared to put her 1970s-like cabaret act in the circus of show-business novelty acts, reminiscent of Jessie Owens racing horses or Sitting Bull parodying his life in Buffalo Bill Cody's Wild West extravaganza.

My own scepticism embarrasses me. I want to believe her. I want to ask the Egyptians what's it like to be a mummy and why they didn't invest in a retirement plan. I beg the Thomas principle: show me some proof. Put me in touch with some of my relations. They are difficult questions, and I get short change. She tells me she can't switch from interview behaviour to what's happening on the other side so easily. I'm not convinced. I ask again. 'If you want, maybe later you could ring my psychic line, but be warned, there's a three-month waiting list.' I bet there is, and I bet there's greenbacks involved too. We wrap as a new shift begins and her PR machine kicks in. 'Don't forget to mention the website address.' I knew she'd say that: psychic or what?

Anyway, that's all in the past, so to speak, and by the time you stand up fully in the toilet (back in the present), the old chute is feeling a little tender. Sore, even. Holding your cheeks together causes some internal discomfort, but it doesn't last. Later on in the day, the tightness comes back. Passing any sort of stool – I'm being polite here – becomes a scourge. 'Jesus,' you say to yourself every second time you go, 'that was painful.' It becomes something to be avoided, which is a bloody shame. Most blokes love the quietness, solitude and happiness of minding your own business sitting in the jacks, reading the paper or just contemplating dinner. In fact, Nathaniel Gubbins, the English writer and journalist, was wrong when he said that 'In that part of the world which is called civilised, there are only three places you can avoid women: the club, the monastery, and the grave'. There is a fourth: the bog. It's the one place in the house where you can just step out of your life for as long as you want. I'm sure that a solitary uninterrupted read in the toilet can take years off a person's life, and that anyone with a dodgy heart would do better to replace a half-hour walk every day with just two twenty-minute me-time sessions in the bog.

Struggling to do what should come naturally to you, you think that maybe it's dietary. Too many carbohydrates, even overdoing the bran, fruit or vegetables. You laugh. Maybe, maybe not. In truth, you haven't a clue. Do you ring up the doctor and make an appointment again? Yes, again. You're already attending for a liver complaint – yeah, fatty liver, as explained earlier in the year, the one that pokes you on your right-hand side – and you've had more than your fair share of flu visits already this year, and there are the continuing difficulties with obesity. Do you really want to call the doctor? He's bound to think: 'Oh, Jesus, it's this hypochondriac again. So what's wrong with you now, a hernia, a sore toe, or are you having trouble sleeping on a bed of nails? Don't tell me: you've had visions.' No, best to see if it goes away.

But it doesn't go away. The presence of blood gets a little more obvious. Passing stools becomes an ordeal out of the Inquisition's top five ways to torture excommunicants, and visits to the loo seem to last for days. You begin to believe you have a blockage, certainly something stopping the easy flow of the unwanted dark stuff. It starts to affect how you drive the car, how you have sex, how you pull weeds, how you talk and converse with your friends. A permanent frown rests on your face as if you cannot explain how you managed to forget what currency you were paid to decorate a house in 1994.

You confide in the wife. She tells you to go to the doctor. You tell her he'll think you're a hypochondriac. She suggests the chemist. *For what?* Ask him has he any suppositories or anus cream. *Me? Are you out of your mind?* Well, it'll help. A couple of suppositories and a rub of anus cream, and you'll have a whole new hole. *Oh, please, will you go for me? I couldn't bear the embarrassment. He'll think there's something wrong with me.* No he won't; he's a chemist. *Yes he will, and the fact that he's a chemist has nothing to do with it.*

And so the Conscience relents, and comes back with enough torpedoes to design, build and blow up the Tower of Babel, and lashings of anus cream. The cream is easy. Rub, rub, rub, and we're in business. Inserting the bloody suppositories twice a day is nearly as unsettling as the problem I'm hoping they'll repair. And getting my fingers in a position to launch the medication is as awkward as playing Twister. Irritated, you want to ring up the games manufacturers and tell them you've invented a game called Solitaire Twister for overweight adults aged twenty-five to fifty, which comes equipped with fourteen towels, 8,096 packets of suppositories, and a mirrored mat fitted with a coat of disinfectant to stand on. OK, so you need a lot of storage to play it, and the cost might be prohibitive, but you'll at least give any sufferer of anus stress the reassurance that they're not the only one who knows about it.

They say the best way to insert suppositories rectally – and even saying the word disturbs me – is to imagine a space between your cheeks, breathe in, push, and allow the space to swallow it. In the morning, hunched awkwardly over the bath at home, twisting my body for maximum effect, anyone going by the bathroom, or more importantly our neighbours, with whom we share a main wall, are bound to think the sounds emanating from the toilet could only be the little fat bloke next door practising for the 105 kg weightlifting class at the Olympic Games.

Anyway, I give it a go. Lots of gos. For whatever reason, the success rate – and I don't want to get too mathematical – was extremely poor. In fact, in fifteen attempts, in the one sitting – it sounds like I was eating them, but I can assure you I wasn't – I couldn't even get one to stay up. By number sixteen, and the second packet, the Conscience lets out a roar: 'Are you finished yet?' The intensity of my fright in itself drove the projectile towards its intended target. A sharp intake of breath later, and I stood up straight and regained my balance. The little white rocket scored a home run, swallowed into the space like your favourite pen would be sucked into a vacuum cleaner. Despite a slight pain and further irritation, and a minute of checking to make sure the bloody thing hadn't fallen out, it was obviously doing its job, a fact borne out by – and I won't dwell on this – the discoloration of my stools an hour later. By the time I was finished, my fingers were thick and discoloured, with the smell of zinc oxide, bismuth sugallate, hard fat and balsam Peru – ingredients I would normally never have heard about, if I hadn't felt the need to read the packet to make sure there wasn't anything in the formula that I needed something stronger than a bar of soap to remove.

*

This went on for about a week, during which time I'm sure I was competing with the whole Chinese nation for the world supply of suppositories, and that I was affecting the commodities market with hedge-fund managers selling oil, gold and the US dollar, and chucking any available excess into suppositories. Anyway, the upshot was that they didn't work.

So, against my better judgement, I went to the doctor. 'Hello, Paul,' says the doc, eyeing me with those narrow, beady irises that touch the eyebrows on their tippy-toes, telling you that he thinks you're a hypochondriac. 'What can I do for you?' 'Bum trouble,' says I, filling him in on what I couldn't get out, at least not without a struggle. A prescription later, for more powerful suppositories – nuclear ones – and enough powdered constipation relief to unplug a battleship, I'm playing have-you-used-these-before? with the chemist, who obviously doesn't remember me from the last time, or does, and just doesn't want to stigmatise me as a serial suppository user. Coming home from the chemist's with boxes up over my head, I'm wishing I lived in a bigger house.

The Conscience, of course, isn't impressed. 'He gave you *how* much?' says she, exasperated by how small her bathroom has become. 'You'll have to put them in the shed. I'd be embarrassed if anyone called and saw them.' (As if she'd show people into the bathroom to say 'And here we have Paul's bum-unblockers'.) 'Like, it's not normal, is it?' That's my wife, all right. I'm wondering if my hole will ever be a hole again, and she's wondering what the family and friends will think if they realise I've a problem around the personal canals. And now that I think of it, she hasn't always been as loyal as I had expected. There was that time when she took all my chocolates away from me and brought them into her work, where she raffled them to her colleagues by asking them to think of a number between one and ten. I found this a bit disturbing. She never asks me to think of a number. But then again, she's often lampooned me to her friends. She was once discussing my weight problem with a friend when the conversation turned to junior rikishis – those poor unfortunates whose chores include wiping the arses of Sumo wrestlers. Says she: 'Jesus, I wonder could I get one of those for Paul for his birthday.' Thanks, love. Solidarity and all that. So much for the helpful soulmate. Bet Nadezhda Krupskaya never said, when Lenin was putting on a bit of weight: 'You'll never guess, Vladimir Ilyich Ulyanov, what I got you for your fortieth?'

Anyway, two weeks later, having lived on constipation-relief powder morning and night, and nearly broke a rib or two contorting my body clockwise so that my fingers could hold and fire the suppositories with some hope of success, it all came to a head – or should I say it *didn't* come to a head. I'm usually regular 6 AM, 8 AM, 12 noon and maybe 8 PM for the big ones, and every half-hour on the hour or half-hour if I'm drinking buckets of water, for the small ones. This day, without thinking about it for a second, I thought it was just going to be the same as usual. The usual early-morning clear-out became a problem almost immediately. It was a full-blown strike. *En grève! En grève! En grève!* the stools seemed to be bellowing. No movement whatsoever, their placards poking reminders somewhere in the impasse. There wasn't even the briefest of hellos. So I sat, and sat, and sat, pushing for dear life, trying to get something to move. Feeling slightly faint from my exertions, I tried to relax. Let nature take its course. Again, nothing. So I got up, had the breakfast, and drank plenty of water. Still nothing. And yet the urge was there to empty every bit of badness through the only exit point that should be listening.

Eventually, eight litres of water later, the banks finally broke, in the most painful discharge I have ever had in my life. 'Aggghh! Aggghh! Aaaaagghh!' I screamed, the stool coming through my hole as if it was a tug-of-war between gravity on the one end and five of the heaviest haemorrhoids somewhere upstream on the other end. 'Agggh! Oh, oh, oh!' I moaned, bouncing on the ceramic for a smidgen of relief, the agony bringing the wife to the door as if I was jumping around like a monkey auditioning for I'm-A-Stool-Get-Me-Out-of-Here. I have never felt pain like it. In fact, if anything was excruciating, this was it. Evil, intense and mind-fucking, it just wouldn't go, lingering on a tripwire along my nerve system, the type of pain you pray someone or something will push off and divert to its death, miles below in the ravine. Minutes later, I had to go again. The intensiveness of this evacuation, if you could teach it to war-on-terror interrogators anywhere in the world, would have anyone who knew where Osama Bin Laden (a man with a great diet who apparently likes bread, yoghurt, honey and dates but rarely eats meat – I look forward to the day when someone asks him for his favourite GI diet) was hiding quickly providing maps, diagrams and nursery rhymes of where he was living, how many times a day he played bingo, whether he shopped in Marks and Spencer, and his travel arrangements for the next twenty years. It was a lingering pain that just wouldn't go away; in fact, it lasted the whole morning. I couldn't talk, walk, jump, sit, sleep, read, listen or paint; the pain broke every rule under the United Nations convention against torture and other cruel, inhuman or degrading treatments or punishments. It was so bad, all I could do was go out and dig the allotment, clearing out with a vengeance any weeds that got in my way.

Obviously I was desperate that I wouldn't have to talk to anyone, putting my head down in as narrow-minded a way as possible to stop the neighbours encroaching. Within six or seven hours, and despite forty-six visits to the toilet – I kept a count, in case the doctor asked me, when I went to see him on the Monday – I had cleared every known family of weed in or around my patch within a depth of two foot. By teatime, the pain in the out-chute had abated, and I could at least sit down.

The following day, Sunday, it was déjà vu, except that I didn't dig the allotment, preferring to moan, both in and out of the bathroom. By Monday morning, I was banging down the walls to the doctor's surgery looking for an appointment. I got an early one. The first thing the doctor says to me is: 'Are you worried you've got colon cancer?' 'Colon cancer?' I say in astonishment. 'I only came in for something for my hole.' He then puts on a pair of rubber gloves as if he's doing his James Robertson Justice impression of Sir Lancelot Spratt, an image that even now gives me the heebie-jeebies. 'Roll up there on the couch and I'll have a look,' he says. 'And be prepared, this is going to be painful.' *Jesus*, I say to myself, *he's enjoying this.*

So up I get, turn on my side, and before I can say 'Can you see anything yet?', he's rammed two of the most vicious fingers in medical history up my out-shute. I scream so loud the doctor closes the window. 'I'm finished,' he says. I want to say, 'Yes, you are, buddy', but I listen instead. 'I think I'll send you to a specialist.' And so a week later I'm lying up on a couch, turned on my side, and the consultant is putting two more of the most vicious fingers in medical history a little more forcibly up my poor hole. 'Jesus! Jesus! Jesus!' I scream, my body nearly rocking the couch through the adjoining wall. 'I think you're not too bad, but you might have a fissure,' he says. I feel as if I'm Jerusalem and that the consultant has just divided my hole in four, giving a portion each to the Armenians, Christians, Jews and Muslims.

By the time I'm walking home like an inhabitant of the Galápagos, I've a prescription for all sorts of procedures, fact sheets explaining everything, multiple instructions, and a hospital appointment for a colonoscopy: hole surgery. Having read what a fissure is – a tear or split in the skin covering the muscle ring of my hole, a sort of sentinel pile – I make my way to the chemist for my medication: glyceryl trinitrate, or GTN, which I'm alarmed to discover later can also be used as an explosive! However, no sooner am I in the local chemist than the pharmacist tells me that glyceryl trinitrate comes only in 0.4 percent preparations and that my consultant has made a mistake, writing 0.2 percent on the prescription. 'Ah,' I say, 'he told me this would happen' – which he did – and that I'm to assure the chemist that 'Yes, 0.2 percent is right.' In fact, he emphasised this by writing the calculation in bold. 'He said, "They'll probably have to dilute it."' 'Dilute it with what?' she asks. 'You tell me. You're the chemist,' I reply, beginning to think I'm not overly comfortable that I should be doing business with this particular apothecary. It's not like I'm a drug-pusher and I'm expecting them to make up soap-bar or formula, and wondering how much used engine oil I should be adding to the ingredients.

She starts foostering around looking in old bin-liners, drawers and medicine cabinets, makes a few phone calls, and scratches her head before giving up and telling me to ring my consultant for the proper percentage. I don't. I go to a different chemist, who tells me to come back the following day and that they'll have 'to mix it up'.

I had been given a whole series of instructions as to how to put the ointment on. Only use a pea-size amount, and make sure you wear gloves. The ointment is absorbed through the skin, and you don't want to overdose. Do not rub it on, but dab it. How the hell do you dab a pea-size amount in the middle of a target you cannot see and can hardly reach? Once applied, try not to wipe it off, which was a polite way of saying 'Go to the toilet first'. Oh, and by the way, headaches are a side effect of 0.2 percent GTN cream in 'almost all cases'. Not surprisingly, within ten seconds of applying the cream, I am cut down with migraines, and for the next eight weeks I become a paracetamol junkie. (I have also been given an ointment to relieve the itch. Did I mention the itch? No? Well, there's another trauma for you – and another ointment, called proctosedyl, which is supposed to work like the bejaysus to reduce the pain, irritation and itching around the back door. This is a side effect of my present condition, which has me making inroads into the EU's toilet-paper mountain. Need I say more?)

It's a lonely furrow, and one that's difficult to explain. It's certainly not something you want to bring up in polite conversation. You ponder why you haven't got a mentor and why you have never been a protégé. I decide to take action. Thus, The I-Was-Never-A-Protégé-Either (IWNAPE) support group was founded by myself and another man whose name I didn't get, somewhere between Broadstone and Glasnevin, upstairs on the 19A bus. At the time it was coming on for eleven o'clock at night, miserably inclement and very dark, and we weren't sure where we were stopped in traffic, when we both realised we had never been protégés. I did most of the talking, while the man agreed with everything I said.

I began by telling him that as a very young child – possibly aged three or four – I was constantly reminded by my own sensibilities that I wasn't loved. By the time I had learned to verbalise my concerns at around five, my mother – who still thinks to this day that she has a sense of humour – suggested buying me a T-shirt inscribed 'Nobody Loves Me', so the world would be aware of my worries. For the next thirty-five-odd years, I have subsequently been the butt of my mother's joke to brothers, sisters, assorted toys, aunts, uncles, neighbours, girlfriends, wife, and every second carpenter, plumber or electrician who ever did work in my parents' house when I was growing up. And so, from a very early age, I concluded that, despite whatever I did in life, and the percentages of happiness that came my way, I would never be truly loved – a fact endorsed by my parents – and that no one would ever come to my rescue or offer mentorial support. In essence, I would never be anyone's protégé. It was at this stage that I had to wake my co-founder, who had fallen asleep before I could elaborate on my time in school.

Early in my education, there appeared to be some hope. My first teacher – who shall remain nameless, more for the fact that I don't want her to know she was right in the end – took an interest in me for some unknown reason, sat me up the front and allowed me to prosper a little. Prospering, for a five-or six-year-old at the time, meant that I was possibly bright and could be excused classes some Friday afternoons, to help the local nuns put out their chairs for a monthly conference over in the opposite wing of the school. For two to three hours' work, I was paid in kind with a chocolate bar. Oh, the innocence of it all. Sadly, in retrospect, it was the nearest I ever got to being a protégé. I bet you that, nowadays, no six-year-old worth his battery-controlled Spiderman would work for anything less than two boxes of chocolates, no homework for a month and an extra day's holiday.

By the time I had made a subsequent move to another school, where apparently I didn't shine, and then on to another school, where I was reunited with my first teacher – who couldn't believe how much I'd changed and told me that at eleven years of age I was a 'complete waster and doomed' – the bus had jerked to a stop amid a cacophony of car-horns, and my new best friend, who had been waiting for quite a while to interrupt me, uttered the immortal words: 'I was never a protégé either.'

'Brilliant,' I replied. 'That's what we'll call our support group.' I then proceeded to recall from memory my undistinguished career at secondary school, in the boy scouts, and at university, my various degrees of failure at sport, and my early adventures in employment. How was it that, despite the thousands of people I have met, no one ever saw me as protégé material? Was it misfortune? Was I not tall enough? Was I ugly? Was I lazy? Or was I just too stupid? Maybe it's one of life's conundrums. All I can say is that, over the years, I've noticed the nods and the winks of outrageous fortune and the hushed tones of 'That's yer man's protégé' or 'That's your woman who's tipped for the big job' as other people walked on my soul, mind and head, metaphorically speaking in all cases but the third, where I have the marks to prove it.

During a lean spell of unemployment in the 1990s, I thought my luck was changing when a supervisor-type plucked me from the dole queue, only to tell me that I'd been overpaid for four months' welfare and would I mind if they recouped their largesse over the subsequent three years at fivepence a week? Obviously I was quickly back in employment, and the debt remains outstanding to this day – until the next time I sign on, I suppose. Even in the hallowed halls of government, my name is probably mud.

As I recalled my tenure in freelance journalism – swapping the sweat on my brow for the spit between my fingers, and wondering how I've ended up battering a keypad for a living, making unintelligible squiggles with my faithful pen while waiting for my faithful editors to return yesterday's calls or to sanction the go-ahead on the three-hundred-odd stories I've got in storage – my nameless friend said 'This is my stop' and 'Sure, we must meet up sometime to discuss what it's like to never have been a protégé', as he quickly scurried down the stairs.

So, there I was – a lonely, unguided Telemachus waiting for the goddess Athena to inspire any semblance of a mentor, an Alcibiades without Socrates, Timothy without St Paul, T. S. Eliot without Ezra Pound, Martin Luther King without Benjamin Mays, or Eminem without Dr Dre – when the busman woke me and told me that the bus had reached the terminus and was I going to get off? Even Dublin Bus doesn't love me.

Anyway, by the time the eight weeks were up, I had applied the 0.2 percent GTN nearly every day, and found myself one morning at half past seven sitting in a smock in a hospital bed waiting to go down to surgery. Two days before, I had started the colonoscopy preparation, which involved a complete clean-out of the waterworks and various canals down below. My consultant had told me to take two Senokot tables at 10 PM two days before the test and strongly advised me to stay within five feet of a toilet. After midnight, I was to take no solids or milk and drink plenty of water and fizzy drinks. At 8 AM on the morning before the test, I dissolved a sachet of Picolax into a glass of water and drank it, followed by another glass of the same mixture at 2 PM. I was warned that it might get hot and bubble up. 'Jesus,' I said to the wife, as I poured the contents into the water. 'Stand back, I don't know how big this thing gets.'

Reading the warning – 'Be prepared for frequent bowel movements within three hours of drinking the first sachet of Picolax' – for a second time, I made sure to put all the morning papers on a stool beside the toilet, reminding my wife that I had booked the room for the day. Over the course of those two days, I probably lost more weight than I'd lost in the previous three months, although the pain I'd had to go through to get there would be reason enough against advising anyone else to choose this as their diet of choice.

So there I was sitting up in the hospital bed waiting for the bum surgery. 'Don't worry,' at least eight nurses and four junior doctors told me – belying the crisis in the health service – 'you won't remember a thing, and by the time it's over, it'll be time to go home.' Like hell I'd forget. Towards the end of the surgery, I woke up screaming, as if the team of doctors was pulling a boa constrictor down my alimentary canals and out through my anus. The pain wasn't in the ha'penny place, although the 'all clear' an hour or two later came as some satisfaction.

Three weeks later, I went back to see the consultant for the three-week check-up. I met with one of his juniors. It was a quick discussion. Says he: 'Has anyone told you about your colon disease?' 'Colon disease, what colon disease?' 'Well, you have divertututututututu . . . icular disease', says he, with his hand over his mouth. 'Sorry, I missed that. Can you repeat it?' Again, with his hand over his mouth, he muttered something like 'Divertututututu . . . icular disease. *Fuck*, I said to myself, *this is just my luck, the doctor's got a stutter, and I'm in very serious danger of saying 'Thank you' and, not wanting to embarrass him, walking straight out of the surgery in complete ignorance.* Probably taking his cue from the confusion lighting up my face, the doctor decided for all our sakes to write it down. On the back of a blank prescription sheet, he drew a diagram and, leading me with a pen, said 'We are here', as if we were Hansel and Gretel and we were going for a walk up my hole with a packet of cola cubes, bon-bons and bulls' eyes. 'This here is your aaaaanus and if you follow the canal up your back passss-age, there are these little poc . . . kets which go nowhere. This is divertutututututututut . . . icular disease, written "d i v e r t i c u l a r d x" ('dx' being some skewed medical abbreviation for disease). Thank you very much and good . . . bye.'

'Steady on a minute', says I. 'What can I do about it?'

'Nothing, it is something you have to li . . . ve with. If you get a fever or severe sss . . . tomach pa . . . in, go to A&E. They'll look after you.' With that, he wrote some more.

'Is that a prescription?' I asked.

'No,' says he, 'it's a web address.'

'A web address?'

'Yes, a web address, you can looook up all about it on the internet.'

With that, his phone rang and he had a discussion with a close friend or lover about what they were going to have for dinner. 'Are we not having chips again? Do you not know any recipes that don't include potatoes?' Apparently, the stutter was only professional. Throughout the little culinary tête-à-tête, the doctor pointed across the table, wagging his finger at me, in that internationally recognised symbol for 'Don't go yet', as if he had something really important to tell me. Getting off the phone, says he: 'Bloody new wi . . . fe, has made c . . . hips for my di . . . nner every day since I mo . . . ved in with her. Now she tells me she's going to make me something different.'

'What's that?' I ask, as it could possibly have something to do with my divertutututututututu . . . icular disease.

'Wa . . . ffles. Bloody wa . . . . .ffles. Anyway, thanks for com . . . ing.'

And that was it, I was off. Diagnosed in sixty seconds, lumbered with a new disease to add to the burgeoning arsenal, and told to look up the internet if I wasn't sure what I had. And in case the Conscience grilled me when I went home about what the doctor had said, I had a personal sketch of my hole written on the back of a blank hospital prescription form, by the Salvador Dali of the medical world. The modern health service, I thought, Irish style.

For the record, diverticular disease (also known as diverticulosis) is a condition of the large intestine whereby small sacs or pouches called diverticula set up home in the wall of the large intestine. These diverticula can become infected, leading to a condition known as divertic, or hole, trouble. Nearly three-quarters of the population will get it at some time or other, generally in old age, although most don't even know they have it. Symptoms? Abdominal cramps and farting. It is said that you can prevent diverticular disease and its complications simply by eating a healthy diet – high-fibre, low-fat, with lashings of fruit, veggies, wholemeal bread and wholegrain cereals – and introducing a bit of exercise, drinking at least two litres of water per day and, no matter who tells you otherwise, staying the bejaysus away from anything with seeds that might wind up the diverticula.

The liver problem, on the other hand, is probably a little more worrying. It is a pain in the right side of my stomach that never goes away. Sitting down at the computer, hammering away at the words or lying to one side on the sofa, a little bulging dagger sticks out from my right side, poking me like a nagging woman. Little darts of discomfort fold into a massive irritation, like a baker kneading aggressively in the folds of his dough for a pencil. There are times when I feel I am the unmade bread fighting with the yeast, begging it not to rise, blowing the air out, battling nature and the obesity that clings to my liver. Getting to sleep at night is increasingly an issue, with my body only comfortable on one side. And driving the car is also a problem, particularly on longer journeys. Fatty liver tissues, I'm told, will go away if I can do something about my diet. This means changing it. The nuclear, life-changing option: give up fatty foods for ever and join the fit-ness-and-salad brigade. I have gone to numerous doctors and I attend the liver clinic every six months, where a different doctor, twice a year, gives the same advice: lose the weight. I'm beginning to imagine that my liver is a township unto itself, getting bigger, each day going a further step down the road to killing me. It's the one worry that might force me to lose the weight.

The problem is that my GP thinks that the pain in my side has nothing to do with my liver, preferring a diagnosis akin to the side effects of being pregnant – which is probably a poor metaphor, considering that I'm a bloke and I couldn't possibly imagine what being pregnant is like. Anyway, according to the GP, apparently the liver isn't the type of organ you'd expect to find at a knife-fight – unlike the one that keeps picking on me, with its dagger-like internal thrusts. No, the poking pain is symp-tomatic of a strain coming from my back. 'Pregnant women get it all the time', I was told. Now, while at times you might think I was pregnant from the look of me, I am still more sceptical than a room full of Thomases. The reason? Well, the pain only affects my right-hand side, never the left.

Just to be sure, though, the GP sent me for a few scans, which all found nothing, strengthening the GP's argument. As for the specialists in the liver clinic, their only response is 'Lose the weight, Paul, right', while at the same time tapping on the space where my liver should be and shaking their heads, as if their years in medical school mean that they don't need to verbalise what's going through their minds. So, just in case, I'm right, and the GP and the whole liver medical world is wrong, and without raising any major flags about my last will and testament, and all the words-of-a-dying-man bullshit, I'd like to put it on record that I think it's something else. Clue? It's the liver, stupid.

Because if I am wrong and the whitecoats are right, that effec-tively gives me one less reason for losing weight. Like, who would be worried about back pain when you're trying to lose weight? Absolutely nobody. Liver pain, now there's something to put the fear of God in you, and reason enough for me to convince the voices in my head around feeding time that I should at least seriously consider the consequences of my habitual overeating.

SEPTEMBER

CHILDHOOD PSYCHOLOGY
OR WHERE DID IT ALL GO WRONG?

I am sure that somewhere in the depths of my unconscious lurks the real reason why I frantically eat the way I do, hysterically taking two steps at a time to mealtimes, constantly fighting the clock, and time, and the food bells that ring and ring, waking me up, putting me to sleep, injecting adrenaline into my dreams, or bell-tolling me to the next nosh-up. Often, for days, I'm panic-buying in my head, running around imaginary shopping centres wondering what I'll have for Friday lunch. It often becomes a quality-of-life issue. Sometimes, I think there's a baby magpie on heroin riding the food-bike in my head, pedalling me from food-nest to food-nest, plundering anything and everything to feed my habit, on an expenses cheque that my quality of life is cashing. Sometimes my condition leads to a gateway that sticks its nose around the corner to Depression-ville – occasionally I am so down that I don't even want to change the calendar in front of my desk – but it quickly turns back, my appetite greater than any melancholy.

Fullness is also not an excuse to the demon inside me. In 'Night Comes On', Leonard Cohen captures the essence of my temptation. Halfway through the song, he says: 'I needed so much to have nothing to touch – I've always been greedy that way.' That, in essence, is my waking and everyday dilemma. I am sure that I am not the only one living with this phantom, nor the only one out of their right mind, waking up every morning thinking of what they are going to eat today, tomorrow or over the following weekend? But maybe that's all getting a little too technical. Maybe there's no prehistoric instinct driving it, and childhood is in fact to blame.

It's difficult to say when I first decided I had it in me to be a fat git, although the signs were always there. From an early age I ate badly but never put on weight. I was probably just too active. When I was in my late teens, I once ran the Belfast City marathon, and rang home to tell my mother that I had finished the course, and that I would be home on the next train – a two-hour journey – followed by a half-hour trip on the bus, and would she mind making me home-made chips to make up for the weight I'd lost. When I arrived home, I ate five large plates of chips, with a half-pound of sausages, if I remember correctly. It was savage, but within the realms of manageability in those days, provided that I didn't stop running. By the time I stopped running, ten or more years later, it cost me probably half a stone annually.

Long before that, when I was a child, my father was probably the first person to mention anything to me about my size. Nothing sinister, you understand. I can still see him joking with me as he slagged me off that I was too thin, to the signature tune: 'Skinnymalink, melodeon legs, umbrella feet.' Not that this made me want to be obese, I'm sure. In fact, if I reminded him of this now, he would still laugh at me, and would probably be right. Nevertheless, my earliest memories of overeating revolve around a serious appetite for chips, particularly home-made chips, and eating entire giant cardboard boxes of Lincoln Creams rejects that my mother bought from someone she knew in the biscuit factory. In those days, we even had a useless biscuit tin that, some day, someone will find buried in our house, minus the family history. For me, it had the same magnetic attraction that would normally draw historians or the religious of Hollywood to the Ark of the Covenant. Every morning, I would sneak down the stairs before anyone was up to raid this little metallic tabernacle. The tin held the two or three packets of biscuits that my mother would have added to the weekly shopping. In many ways, my mother was my co-conspirator in this adventure. If she hadn't opened every packet of biscuits into the tin in the first place, in some misguided belief that the biscuits would be kept fresher out of their wrappers and within the confines of the biscuit jar, I wouldn't have had a youngster's confidence to dig in with gusto. Like, how many biscuits are in a packet? Even an adult doesn't know. Would my mother miss three, four or five? I doubted it: it was going to be a biscuit-fest. It was easy to count eight biscuits and take three from each packet. If there were three packets, I would easily have nine biscuits for myself. Ironically, it was like taking biscuits from a child, although I wouldn't have necessarily thought of that at the time. I was more your indiscriminate biscuit-bandit, and not particularly academic. If I'd been around when Niall had the nine hostages, I would have been known as 'O'Doherty of the Nine Biscuits'.

Anyway, by the time the big brown cardboard boxes of Lincoln Creams cast-offs arrived, it may as well have been the California Gold Rush, to my mind. I immediately discarded what was left of the biscuit tin. I was in the big league now, and keen to eat my way through my very own *Treasure of the Sierra Madre*. It was possibly what you might call the beginning of my fool's gold, the march to obesity. But sitting there in the early morning in my pyjamas, the world was a happy place, and all I could see were the hundreds, if not thousands, of Lincoln Creams that were stacked twenty-five or thirty high and ten or twelve (or was it fourteen?) abreast. Jesus, I must have thought to myself, I could take as much as I want, and they'll never know I've been here, ever. I probably even saw my name up in shiny lights: *The Ghost Biscuit-Bandit Rides Again* – starring Flash Gordon Zorro Trampas O'Doherty.

Looking back on it now, I must have woken every morning at the crack of dawn, for a month, and run down that stairs with enough momentum to drag any number of classifiers, highbankers and gold-pans, and all the other gold-prospecting paraphernalia needed to keep me in the biscuit-hills for years. I would have been happy to bury my heart at wounded knee, my life's childish ambitions already fulfilled.

Despite this mindset, it didn't take long for the Lincoln Creams heist to come to light, and before I had time to escape to

Brazil or anywhere else that didn't have an extradition treaty with my mother and father, I found myself locked in my room from dusk until dawn – although my mother has always denied this. Years later, she told me that she locked me in my room because she was afraid that my younger brother would get out of bed in the middle of the night, open the bedroom door, go for a walk and fall down the stairs, or do something awful like mill into the Lincoln Creams – which in fairness probably worried me as well. That, however, doesn't explain the number of times – and they were considerable – when I was locked in my room on my own as a form of punishment. It was a lonely, brutal existence that drove me crazy with anger, so much so that, years later, my parents had to replace the bedroom door because I had chiselled through the locks with an Action Man's right hand – as good as any rock-hammer you would find in Shawshank. To be fair-minded to my parents, it was probably never as bad as I remember it, and they certainly didn't tie me to a radiator or anything like that.

Lincoln Creams aren't a kick-in-the-arse away from being shortcake biscuits – which I love with nearly as much as a passion as home-made chips – with their mad little concentric circles of dots. My mother used to put me on her knee and sing to me Mama's Little Baby Loves Short'nin' Bread, along with other nursery rhymes like Pat a Cake, Pat a Cake; Jack Sprat; Jack be Nimble; Tom, Tom, the Piper's Son; There Was an Old Woman; Simple Simon; Little Tommy Tucker; Sing a Song of Sixpence; Pop Goes the Weasel; and Peter, Peter, Pumpkin Eater. My mother, as you can make out, seemed to have an obsession with feeding me on a diet of nursery rhymes that either involved the preparation, baking, eating of or begging for food. What was I to do – I was a baby? I couldn't turn around and say, 'Jaysus, Ma, can you cut us a little slack with the fucking nursery rhymes. I think you're going to cause irrecoverable damage to my developing psyche and I'll be left with a chip and biscuit obsession for the rest of my life'. For this reason, some judge somewhere should be honour bound to find nursery rhymes just as dangerous as victim impact statements. There is psychological research somewhere on the effects and benefits of reading nursery rhymes to the unborn child in the womb, and it's quite staggering. Apparently, a child who has heard particular nursery rhymes in the womb will have a preference for hearing them again when they are born, over ones they never heard in the womb. I suspect this is probably one of the reasons why civil war politics has existed in Ireland for so long, with mothers and fathers up and down the country, far too openly discussing the Fianna Fáil ard fheis or why Fine Gael is a yo-yo party in full hearing of the foetus. Like, sure no wonder Sinn Féin hasn't made a proper breakthrough in the South in the last twenty-five years. When all those mothers should have been in singing Republican rhymes to their babies in their wombs, they were instead outside the front door banging those drums in favour of Hunger Strikers or against the RUC.

Out of nappies and about to start school, food had a sort of routine in those days. Monday was leftovers, obviously from Sunday, and if there wasn't enough, some sort of a coddle, usually with potatoes, sausages and rashers, was added. Tuesday was mince at my Auntie Kay's in Walkinstown, in the company of my cousins Ann and Debbie. Wherever we lived, whether it was in Ballymun or Clondalkin, we made the journey by bus or car to Dublin 12 for mince every Tuesday of my life (excluding holidays and Christmases). Wednesday, as I have pointed out earlier, was fish and home-made chips. Thursday was a springer, and we never knew what we were going to get, although in winter it was invariably stew or, if we went to my Granny Doherty's, chips. Friday was again fish and chips. My mother was patient to the core on those days, standing for hours on end making chips – some lightly cooked, others a little more finished and crispy – until the family had all been served. Being Friday, it was also a day of abstinence. Abstinence in the sense that we ignored meat and dug into the rock salmon, mackerel or whiting, while my mother served herself plaice, a fish we youngsters were considered too young to appreciate – or maybe that's just a childish memory skewed by time.

Saturday was a fry, and Sunday was either a roast joint (lamb, beef or chicken) or boiled ham, or tongue in a big pot of cabbage.

I hated boiled cabbage. It was one of the first vegetables I could never get my head around – an awful predicament for a young carnivore. My life-long hatred of all things vegetable until my early thirties was born at this stage, during what Piaget calls the 'concrete and the formal' stage. Not surprisingly, I now like my vegetables cooked al dente. My parents believed that the most important ingredient in cooking vegetables was water, using an old Aquarian technique that translates as: 'Boil the bejaysus out of it.' Watery cabbage, watery carrots or watery Brussels sprouts – take your pick. I still have flashbacks of being forced to finish my dinner on Sunday afternoons, looking down on vegetables in need of resuscitation from the cold, and the water being forked around the plate as I try to dodge a food execution. Tom Cruise thought he was brave eating placenta: I'd like to see him eat my mother's watery cabbage. Some scientists even believe it is a cure for Scientology.

Going back to fish days, my mother had a bit of a fetish for plaice, while around the same time, my parents also believed that children weren't big enough to eat choc ices, and so on Sunday-afternoon drives in the car, we sat in the back with a poxy orange ice pop each while the Gestapo sat in the front, licking their chocolate ice creams to death. It was a classic Oedipus scenario, where, on those long, meandering weekend drives in the Wicklow mountains or along the north County Dublin beach front, a young monster with a lollipop sat in the back of the car eyeing his dad with contempt, wondering would his mother buy him a choc ice if he murdered his father.

My primary-school career is also etched on the what-went-wrong board. From the very first day, I was sent to school with banana sandwiches. From aged five to around seven, I lived on banana sandwiches as my packed lunch of choice. I ate so many of them I could have been Potassium Man. In the schoolyard every day, as I ate what kept me regular, one of the nuns there, a notorious battleaxe, went around the playground checking the bins for bread-crusts. She had the same twisted face and heart as the centurion in *Ben Hur* who scolds the Jesus-figure for offering Ben Hur some water, after he has specifically forbidden it. One day, when I was seven, she told me that she had seen me throwing my crusts into the bin, which was a lie. She insisted that I pick the crusts out of the bin and eat them. Even in those days, I am sure that my mind rattled with the obvious: Will I fuck? However, what was OK to think wasn't acceptable to say, so I allowed my politeness to sway me. In my seven-year-old shorts, I told her that I for one wouldn't be pulling crusts out of a bin for no one, particularly when I for one didn't throw them in there in the first place. This resulted in a little bit of an altercation, and my mother was called to the Crucible to defend little Pauly against a possible death penalty for throwing crusts into the witch's bin. Luckily, the old nun having preserved the crime scene and gathered up the offending bread crusts, my mother was able to say under cross-examination that, in fact, she didn't make my lunch from the type of bread that the nun had retrieved. In answer to the charge that I wasn't being accused of throwing a particular type of crust into the bin but the crusts the nun held in her hand, my mother was unequivocal: 'You don't know Pauly. If it's not his, or he's not familiar with it, not only will he not eat it, he won't even touch it.' Case dismissed.

From then on, I knew that my days of eating banana sandwiches were coming to an end. Not long after this incident, I gave up bananas – and banana sandwiches – for life. To this day, I can't stand anything that's either made from, or involves, bananas. Was the nun to blame? Is it a psychological trauma from that day in school? Maybe. Whatever the truth, my mother's assessment that under no circumstances did I touch, never mind eat, anything that I wasn't completely familiar with was, for the most part, true. Unusual sauces, toppings, dips, vegetables, fruit, pastas and curries, among many, many other things, were verboten to my sensibilities and palette, and no amount of coaxing was ever going to change my position. Stubbornness wasn't in the Ha'penny Place.

When we visited relations, neighbours and family friends, they were faced with the perennial what-will-he-eat? dilemma, as they tried their best to convince me that I would love onions or cabbage if I gave them a try, or that I really had nothing to fear from scrambled eggs or runny cheeses. Often, going to family get-togethers was disastrous, particularly if the set meal involved a cold tea that lacked any imagination or goodies. I was once so hungry at one of these gatherings that I bit the glass I was supposed to be drinking from; an incident that embarrassed my parents no end. They have consequently never let me forget it. You can see how my parents were the type of people who would give you a complex. I often thought that the FAI should have approached them years ago about providing one – a complex, I mean.

By the time I was ten, no matter where I went, I had left sensible food way behind me. All I wanted to eat was sweets, chocolate, cake and biscuits. Was I any more abnormal than other kids? I suspect not. Once, around the same time, my mother and father went away and I stayed with my mother's mother. During that week, I was enrolled in a summer school locally; it involved bringing what the flyers sent home to my parents referred to as a packed lunch. Now, ever since I had said goodbye to the banana sandwiches, the notion of a packed lunch was a joke to me. So I set off down the village to do my supermarket shop for my five days in holiday camp. By the time I got there, I was the only one in the shop, and thinking *This will be great and sure I'll be no time*, only to realise at the checkout that they were closed and that I wasn't going to get anything, and would I mind 'coming back at nine in the morning'. The manager then kindly asked me – me being a kid and all that – would I mind putting the assorted biscuits, crisps and minerals back on the shelves. I told him that, seeing as I was going to have to come back at nine in the morning, I could do it then. This didn't go down very well, and the manager pointed to the door with a cartoon character's vulgarity. The following morning I hadn't the nerve to go back to the shop and ended up buying sub-standard rubbish in a grocer closer to where I was staying. It was a mistake I have never willingly made since, buying or stealing – the latter obviously only in my youth – from reliable suppliers.

One such supply line arrived from an unlikely source. A favourite aunt of mine once brought my mother home a present of a tin of Quality Street sweets from a visit to Lourdes – yeah, I know, I can't figure it out either – which my mother promptly hid away for Christmas. On one of my regular childhood scavenging missions around the house and under the mother's bed, looking for anything I could eat, I discovered the miracle of the tin of Quality Street. Carefully removing the Sellotape that ran around the rim of the tin, and delicately hanging the see-through tape from the windowsill – so that I could reseal the tin with impunity – I tucked in, overcome with myself that a casual hunt for the odd Penguin or cheap packet of biscuits had resulted in a mini-lottery. What's great about those large tins of sweets is that you could take out ten or twenty sweets initially and no one would be any the wiser. And after that, you can go back and forth and take out two at a time, and if the worst comes to the worst and you're forced to hand the tin around in company, it's pretty difficult to notice that the Biscuit Bandit's paid a visit. It's nearly as good a trick as the one with the five loaves and two fishes. In fact, I used to wind up my mother by saying that I was sure that, if Our Lord had handed around a tin of Quality Street to the hungry multitude, his miracle would never have got into the papers, because everybody would have said: 'Ah, come off it, Jesus, you can get loads out of one of those tins.'

When my father took down the tin at Christmas, there were only two sweets left. Questioned by the food police for days, my only defence was that, if you take only two sweets every time you go to the tin, you'd be bloody surprised how quickly you make your way through the whole lot. It's all part of the principle behind delusion: if you can delude yourself, you think you can convince others. Although, if I was to be purely cynical, you would have to wonder who brings a tin of Quality Street home from Lourdes in August expecting them to last until Christmas. Like, you would nearly be expecting a miracle, wouldn't you?

Anyway, all in all, this is just another case of my selfish bloody greed. Whatever's inside me, I'm unable to stop taking my share, and everybody else's, at the same time. When I was small, and my brothers and sister were smaller and didn't know any better, every Easter I would carefully remove the tin-foil wrapper on their Easter eggs, eat the sweets inside and wrap the egg up again. Obviously, being little squeaks of kids, they were only too delighted to get chocolate eggs at all; they didn't realise that there were supposed to be sweets on the inside as well.

Like many a parent, my mother did her Christmas-biscuit shopping earlier in the year, and then stashed away the biscuit tins, hoping that I wouldn't find them. But of course I found them. What would you expect, searching in a three-bedroom house in suburbia: that I wouldn't find them? Other than up in the attic, in the parents' bedroom, or in between the coats in the cloakroom, there are not many places left. And you'd be surprised how many parents still hid their food valuables under the bed. It would make you wonder for that generation. My mother once tried to be innovative and hid a box of chocolates in the washing machine, and then forget about them when it came to putting on the week- ly white wash. And, yes, dark chocolate does run. I was popular that week, I can assure you. Blamed for a crime I hadn't commit- ted, I knew exactly how Hannibal and the A-Team felt.

Anyway, getting back to the box of biscuits I found, not sur- prisingly, under my parents' bed, and carefully removing the Sellotape wrapping once again, I took my pick of all the best bis- cuits first, before going on to the second-best and, ultimately, the rest. Even for a kid so young, I had an inherent understanding that, in those days, if there was a biscuit or two missing, the bis- cuit manufacturer was more likely to be blamed for leaving the consumer short than a ten-year-old boy. The problem was that I didn't know when to stop – until, having taken a biscuit from every column in the layer, it was obvious that someone had been 'in'. In desperation, I would rearrange the way they were stacked, putting the bigger biscuits into the smaller holes and vice versa, or placing a big biscuit at the bottom and a small one on top, and any amount of other dodges. I, of course, was banking on the Christmas bedlam, when whoever opened the tin of biscuits – my mother, in most cases – would be so rushed off her feet that she wouldn't have time to realise that the top layer had been rearranged by the resident Biscuit Bandit.

Come Christmas one year, I hadn't reckoned on my mother realising that she hadn't a present for my aunt, who had brought home the box of Quality Street from Lourdes. And so, as a last-minute measure, my mother, when we paid the annual festive visit, gave her a tin of Afternoon Tea biscuits for her Christmas present. I am sure you can see a pattern for eccentricity in our family when it came to exchanging presents. My family could go to the moon for their holidays and they'd likely bring you back a tin of biscuits or a jar of sweets. Of course, I was oblivious to this crazy Christmas present-exchange, right up to the moment my mother handed my aunt a square-shaped object covered in wrapping paper. The shape of the present gave me a shock – an astonishment that was confirmed when my aunt rapped what seemed like a hollow tin on the top and asked: 'Gosh, I wonder what's inside?' This was probably one of the only times in my life when I was terrified for my life. If this had happened in my own home, I would have been sent to bed for a week or docked pocket money, or my mother would have attacked me with the wooden spoon – her weapon of choice – a punishment and minor beating I would easily have accepted in the circumstances. However, public humiliation when you're ten is quite another story.

So there I was, watching my aunt ripping off the Christmas paper and then peeling back the tape on the tin, a nervous wreck, hoping against hope that this was not the tin I thought it was. But of course life is never that easy, and by the time the tin had been passed from my aunt to my uncle, and on again, someone wondered: 'Why are there no chocolate biscuits in the top layer?' Now this is the moment when you pray that your mother will tenderly tap you on the cheek and say: 'Wake up, son, you'll be late for school.' It doesn't happen: the nightmare is coming charging down the track like a train suffering from St Vitus' Dance. Someone else suggests checking the bottom layer. A bomb may as well have gone off. 'Jesus, the bottom layer's empty.' 'Paul!' The roar goes up, and any amount of protestation that 'You should bring them back to Jacobs and get your money back' falls on deaf ears, and the perennial joke is born that Paul – with no consideration for the fact that I was only ten years old at the time – cannot be trusted around biscuits. Not surprisingly, the joke only goes one way, and still elicits a bit of after-burn. Whenever I ask my mother, 'Hey, Ma, how old was I when I did the job with the biscuits?' she quickly responds with the usual: 'Don't you dare ever mention that tin of biscuits!'

Not that that was my only Christmas conviction. When I said I'm passionate about chips and shortbread, I forgot to mention that my third great indulgence is almond icing. I have always loved it, I suppose since I first tasted Christmas cake. Not that I have always been a lover of Christmas cake in itself; that came much later. In the early days, I would sell you all the butter and royal icing it would take to make a thousand cakes – and my soul – for one crumb of almond icing. To my mind, it's a great little delicacy. However, the almond-icing obsession took me as usual below the acceptable level of decency when, years ago, after my mother had carefully rolled out a thick layer of almond icing and attached it to her Christmas cake, I stepped into the equation. It was late November and, following her regular recipe, my mother covered the cake in greaseproof paper and put it away behind the sitting-room sofa – what the recipe deemed, if I remember, a cool, safe spot.

About a week later, I got a touch of the munchies and, finding absolutely nothing of value worth secretly eating in the house, came across the Christmas cake in its shallow hiding place. Bringing it to the kitchen table and having carefully taken off all the greaseproof paper, I removed the almond icing and took the rolling pin to it, rolling it out much thinner than my mother had originally designed. Needless to say, I was able to save a good quarter, and duly ate it, having re-attached the almond icing once again to the Christmas cake, put it back in its greaseproof paper and replaced it under the sofa in the sitting room. It was so beautiful, I repeated the trick five times in the run-up to Christmas and was never caught. It was a great trick, and I subsequently did the same manoeuvre for the next three years, until the mother realised that the almond icing on the Christmas cake wasn't shrinking, and that the finger of blame could be pointed fairly at the Biscuit Bandit. My demise came about when, like all the great greedy people in the world, I got careless, and left a piece of icing on the countertop, not having properly cleaned the crime scene. When my mother found it, she knew instinctually what had happened and, finding the Christmas cake nearly bald a week from Christmas, sequestrated my assets – actually, two weeks' pocket money – to pay for the damage. A confession later, the tale was added to all the other family stories that, essentially, tell the parable of the infamous Biscuit Bandit.

During my years eleven to twelve, I didn't really grow, and certainly didn't put on any weight that would betray that I was a Biscuit Bandit or suffering from a chip obsession. I was very thin, thought I was taller than I actually was, and imagined myself as a handsome devil to boot. By the time I was thirteen, I had caught a glimpse of myself in a mirror or a window, and realised for the first time that I was much smaller than I thought I was and a lot more rounded, although I was not carrying an ounce of fat. Playing all sorts of sports – soccer, rugby, Gaelic and hurling for a time – I was fit, even for my age, if not super-fit. These were the years I could run off any over-indulgence that continued to come my way, despite, even in those days, really loving my food. I once ran away and came home for my dinner: the ignominy of it. I bet you Tom Sawyer or Huckleberry Finn never ran away and came back for their dinner. It's ironic that I have been trying to run away from food ever since.

In those days, my mother used to say: 'Paul, you'll eat me out of house and home.' She never thought to call me a cockatoo; in Australia, these birds have been known to eat houses (not whole houses, you understand, but more than their fair share of the building materials). On some Australian golf courses – God knows what they could eat on a golf course – they even have plastic snakes to frighten the cockatoos away. The cockatoos presumably are afraid of snakes and don't know the difference between a python and a stupid replica with a painted tongue.

Even the church didn't escape my appetite when I was young. From the age of around twelve, I was trained as an altar boy during my religious phase. Coming into the cold, ultra-clean sacristy when it was my turn (there was a rota among the altar boys), often on my own, and having skipped breakfast, the temptation to dig into the unblessed hosts – the thin, wafer breads, that is – was too much for me, once I had set the altar, opened the Bibles on the appropriate pages and lit the candles. As prompt as a shop of clocks, with everything in place, I filled the chalice with the wafers, took a bundle for myself, and then secured the chalice in the tabernacle on the altar. It was a simple routine. Munching on the wafers, I waited for the priest, who lived next door to the church and who had his own entrance to the sacristy. The priest at the time was so regular, in more ways than one, that you could set your clock by him. Every morning he went to the loo, then flushed the toilet and had a deep grunt before entering the sacristy. He never failed to do this, until one morning, while I was divvying out my share of the wafers, he entered the sacristy, taking me by surprise. I quickly chucked the wafers into a plastic bag in which I brought my alb – my vestments – to the church every morning. The priest knew by my actions that I was probably up to no good. 'Paul, don't lie to me. Tell me what you were doing when I came in the door?' I lied, instinctually. 'Nothing, just picking up a pencil I dropped, that's all.' He didn't believe me, but he had no time to quiz me further: he had a Mass to perform.

By the time the Mass was over, the priest said nothing more to me, and we went our separate ways. I was sure that was the last I would hear about it, and I returned to class. Each morning, I got a handy hour off to serve Mass – when it was my turn, you understand – the school being next door to the church. The following morning, I carried the plastic bag with my alb and my schoolbag over the same green I walked every day to and from school; a short hundred-yard distance. As usual, I got off classes at half nine to serve Mass. I did everything I normally did, except that, not wanting to push my luck, I decided to give the wafers a miss, just in case someone above had witnessed my behaviour and felt compelled to dish out some Old Testament-style retribution. Unfortunately, my Catholic conscience was prophetic. No sooner was Mass about to start than two of my neighbours came into the sacristy, which the priest and I was were just about to leave for the altar. Says one of my neighbours, holding up her hands like she was Oliver looking for porridge, with one thin wafer of church bread that was developing a slight green hue in her hands: 'Father, Father, look Father, we found Our Lord lying on the grass outside our house, will He be all right?' *Will He be all right? Jesus,*

171

I said to myself, *will I be all right? The priest will fucking kill me.*
'Thank you very much,' said the priest and, looking over at me,
putting two and two together from the previous morning, said:
'It's probably not consecrated, nothing to worry about.' When
they were gone, he turned down to me like a Tyrannosaurus Rex
picking up his prey: 'Paul, I'll have a word with you after Mass.'
By this stage, I had realised that there was a tiny hole in the end
of my alb bag and that the wafer had squeezed itself through it
like a proper anti-Christ, and landed on the green right outside
my neighbour's house – and me in trouble. *Transubstantiation me
bollix*, I said to myself.

Not surprisingly, this was the longest Mass I have ever attended. Straight after Mass, as the priest was about to hear confessions, he asked me to stay back for a few minutes. Nodding, I took
my opportunity and dashed into the confession box. 'Bless me,
father, for I have sinned,' I began, the sweat forming beads on my
forehead. 'These are my sins. I stole hosts from the box in the sacristy and I am really, really sorry.' Taken aback, the priest gave me
five Hail Marys and five Our Fathers, and out I went. Back in the
real world, and after five other confessions, I asked the priest
when he came out of the confession box did he still want me for
anything? 'No,' says he, 'bit of a misunderstanding. See you in the
morning.' And off I went in the morning, promising never to eat
hosts again, religion, or the fear of it, having cured one food
obsession. Is there a religious cure for my obesity? If there is, I
think I'm long since past it.

Not long after my experiences with the hosts, I was unlucky
enough to get an abscess on my right leg, high up on the inside of
my thigh. At the time, I thought it was divine intervention: a punishment for either stealing the host in the first place or for cun-
ningly confessing the crime without proper conscience to the
priest. The abscess, I was told by the doctor, was 'a right one to
get', whatever the bejaysus that meant, and was caused by either
a splinter or some other form of bacteria that hadn't been properly treated. The upshot of everything was that a cavity had formed
under the skin of my thigh, where pus was gathering for a good
old fight and was now pushing its armies out through my skin as
a defensive mechanism to thwart the infection. For me looking

down on my thigh, it seemed as if I had two penises: one where it should be, and another monstrosity where it shouldn't be, full of primal pus that needed a good kick in the bollocks to get it out in a hurry. So, after the swift visit to the doctor, I was hospitalised while they waited for my infection to come to a head. Close to the time I was due to go down for surgery, the nurse on the ward put a sign over my bed – FASTING – and told me that I wasn't to have anything to eat or drink until after the operation. This was a real bugbear to carry, and feeling that I, and I alone, had been singled out for brutality, I took the sign off the hook over my bed and hung it up over the young fella next to me, who was sound asleep. 'Hail the King of the Jews', it read to me. I thought to myself, *this should be fun.* Of course, when dinner was served, the young fella kicked up a fuss when he woke up, complaining that he wasn't aware that he was fasting and that he should be fed because he was hungry. One of the catering staff had to restrain him, while another went for a nurse. Meanwhile, next door, so to speak, I ate his dinner with gusto.

By the time the nurse came, I had licked the plate clean. Realising what had happened, the crier got his dinner while the nurse turned to me in a temper: 'You're supposed to be fasting. What are you doing eating dinner?'

'I was hungry,' I protested innocently, which didn't seem to assuage the nurse.

'Oh, don't worry,' says she, 'you'll pay for this.'

Pay for it? I thought to myself. *Now that I'm satisfied, how could I possibly pay for it?*

Three hours later, I found out all right, when, with the pus having come to a head, I was taken down to surgery without any anaesthetic. With two nurses holding me down, a doctor asked me if I recognised the painting on the wall. By the time I'd answered 'What painting?' and looked back, the doctor had lanced the apex off my abscess like you'd cut the top off an egg, and then the three of them took turns holding me down, while the other pushed enough pus out of the top of my thigh to fill a bath. Was it painful? You bet your last dollar it was. Would I ever do what I did again? Definitely not. Another useless cure in the long line towards obesity.

OCTOBER

THE MARATHON

In the weeks before the Dublin City Marathon, my option to run hung by a thread. Although I had registered for the race earlier in the year on the off chance that I might be capable of putting in enough training to get me around the course, I hadn't given the event any serious consideration. And if I'm being brutally honest, I had forgotten that I'd signed up in the first place, until, in the middle of October, decision-time came ringing at the end of a phone-line. Even then, the magnitude of what I was deciding never really set in, and I suppose I took the final decision very lightly. With a week left to the event, I made up my mind to give it a go, realising that I wasn't even fit enough to walk to the shops, never mind complete a stamina-sapping marathon. Nevertheless, I stupidly cut out six months of what is generally accepted to be the preparation period for a marathon, putting to the sword, as it were, proper training, exercise and stamina, and hoping to God that pure ability and gutsy will-power would be enough, or, as I said to my wife: 'I am going to do it, and that's the end of it.'

What really kick-started the weeklong training programme was the need to resuscitate a book I was writing: this book. Back in January, in a moment of bravado, I let rip that 'Sure, wouldn't it be great if in the last chapter I ran the Dublin City marathon' – as if you could take a powdered fat bloke, add water, and run a marathon ten months later. I was then an 18-stone monster with a mission – when I wrote a small column in the *Irish Times* called 'An Irishman's Diet' – tying together the various threads, thoughts and nightmares of an ordinary guy trying to lose weight, who was dying slowly in the graveyard of obesity, and feeling it was time to do something about it.

The writing angle was novel. Usually most people hide their diets under their pillows, confessing to having given up the chocolate when the weight police tell them, 'You're looking well', or when they ask, astonished, 'My God, have you lost weight?' I went in the opposite direction: I told everybody I was on a diet and then posted it in the paper. Nailed on like Luther's ninety-five theses. Along the way, Liberties Press came on board, and bang, *An Irishman's Diet* got a book deal. It sounds easy when you say it fast, and everyone at the time thought it was a great idea. I quickly forgot it until, with about ten days to go to the big day, and behind with the book – and when I say behind, I mean a *long* way behind – and wondering would I ever get it finished, the publishers rang to wish me good luck.

'Good luck with what?'

'The marathon.'

'The marathon? Oh yeah, the marathon.'

Lamb of Divine Jaysus, the marathon.

Not one to ignore a challenge, I jumped on a bus immediately after putting the telephone down and went into town and bought the dearest pair of runners – and, no, I don't call them trainers – for €180. Not that this was the first time I have paid over the odds to protect my feet. Once, in my younger days, long, long before the Conscience was on the scene, I had to go out one Saturday and buy a pair of shoes on the morning of a friend's wedding, where I was the groomsman. With a broad pair of feet, getting a pair of shoes to fit was never going to easy. What I didn't realise was that it wasn't going to be cheap either. Anyway, with the clock ticking towards the wedding, I had to shell out £120 for the only pair of black shoes that would remotely fit me. Now, this wouldn't be worth mentioning if it wasn't for the fact that, three weeks after the wedding, when making sure I was getting my money's worth and going everywhere in the runners, I found myself walking this girl home one night. As luck would have it, she invited me in to her parents' house, long past a respectable time when both of us should have been tucked into our own beds. Anyway, keeping our voices to a hush, and making sure not to wake her mother and father, I took off my shoes to give my feet a bit of a breather.

An hour or two later, having said goodnight to the girl, and having put my shoes back on, I left. At home, just before getting into bed, I happened to look down, and noticed the bejaysus of all bejaysuses. I was wearing two odd shoes. Christ, I said to myself, how the fuck did that happen? Now, not one to lose the cool too easily, I put the experience down to drink, made my way upstairs, threw both shoes into the bottom of my wardrobe and went to bed, sort of convincing myself that 'Sure I'm half-pissed and it'll all reveal itself properly in the morning'. Waking up a couple of hours later to go to work, I made a beeline for the wardrobe. No, no, no, I said to myself, recognising in the cold sober morning my own poor unfortunate shoe missing its twin, now nestled with an inferior impostor from God knows where.

Not knowing the girl's phone number or where she worked, and scared shitless to knock on her door, in case someone else answered, I decided to do nothing and put the missing shoe down to the bad luck that has scourged me my whole life. Like, what do you say in those circumstances if you go knocking on someone' door: 'Sorry, but did you happen to find a rather expensive shoe when you were doing the hoovering?'

That was until, a couple of nights later, my mother went berserk while telling me 'There's a woman at the door claiming you have her husband's shoe'. *Oh Christ*, I said to myself, rushing out by her and up the stairs to get the odd shoe. By the time I came down, a woman who I'd never seen before was standing in our doorway pointing my shoe at me, while a man outside our gate in his car gave me a look that had me thanking the bejaysus he hadn't come to the door himself. Exchanging shoes as if we were foreign spies at Checkpoint Charlie, the woman rapped me on the knuckles with my wandering shoe as she left, warning me: 'I hope that's all you left behind.' *Me too*, I said to myself. *Me too, missus*.

Getting back to the marathon, yes, I was paying big bucks for the runners, considering that I only really needed them for one day plus a bit of training, but they had enough shock absorption to get me through at least the first six miles and two-hundred-odd yards in comfort. That only left the other twenty miles to train for. A bit of an Everest, you might say – and you'd be right. Out of my fucking mind? Two out of two. Want to go for a treble? Could I possibly kill myself trying to finish a bloody book by doing something irresponsible and stupid? Bang on, three in a row. With a hit rate like that, one of us should be in therapy.

I went back to the gym and, going against a library of medical books and journals, doctors' advice, and my poor wife's tears, I did what I do best: I embraced the selfish don't-give-a-fuck gene that riddles my DNA by putting my health, and myself and my wife's future, on the line in order to finish the writing of a long-overdue chronicle of a year supposedly on the weight-wagon. It seemed important to me. Since Christmas I had lost about a stone, was fitter than I had been and was definitely eating a lot better, at least most of the time. And over the last ten months, although suffering from a sciatica problem that refused to go away, I had exercised more often than I had for years. I wasn't Eamonn Coghlan but I wasn't Ironsides either.

A week before the marathon, I was tipping the scales at around seventeen and a half stone when my training began. Up in the gym, I cycled ten kilometres on a bike for twenty-five minutes, followed by a five-kilometre, forty-minute walk-cum-run, and ended with ten minutes of stretching. Surprisingly, my back held up, I didn't get that knuckle-like abrasive pain that usually burrows into the left cheek of my bum, and I felt pretty OK. The only problem I experienced was some dizziness immediately after training – this was worrying – and a numbing headache that lasted from the Friday until about seven miles into the marathon on the Monday. Otherwise, for seven days I went to the gym and followed this simple regime.

It amazes me how much planning people put in to running or walking 26.2 miles of what can sometimes be complete and utter boredom. For instance, camouflaging yourself so you're not recognised is up there with wearing the proper running gear, socks and runners, drinking plenty of water, and anointing yourself with enough creams in the crevices that tend to dry up first.

My biggest concern was not being recognised while running like a pregnant bear by peers, friends or, worst of all, enemies. Worse still, I didn't want to be pointed out as running a lousy time. It's fine if you finish in a time of in or around three hours; there's a bit of glory to be found in crossing the line within an hour or so of those who run in the tailwind of the elite runners. Down the pecking order, past the four- and five-hour wasters, comes the ignominy of keeping ahead of what the French call in the Tour de France the *voiture balai*, or the 'broom wagon', which sweeps up the participants who, through injury or fatigue, are unable to continue.

On the morning of the race, and knowing how bloody unfit my body was for a marathon, my heart, body and soul weighted down with imponderables, my biggest concern was whether to wear my prescription shades or my ordinary glasses. I garnered from the weather forecast that it was going to be overcast for most of the day, although I wasn't to be surprised if the odd ray of sunshine shone through. This was a reasonable argument for wearing sunglasses, I thought. However, not quite knowing how fit I was, and predicting the worse, it was possible that I wasn't going to finish the race before it got dark. Would I be able to see in the dark with my sunglasses? Probably not. In the end, the closing argument secured it. I decided that it would be better to wear the prescription sunglasses and have no one recognise me, and chance the experience in the dark, than to run with my ordinary glasses and everyone recognising me as their little fat friend who was writing a book, soon. You'll probably be surprised to hear that even fat people can be vain.

And so, having ignored my wife's repeated pleas for a late but dignified withdrawal, I was standing on the starting line at five to nine in Nassau Street, Dublin, wondering if I would finish the race. Serious premonitions had consumed my weekend, and in the darkest reaches of my mind I sensed that I was in the middle of a gunfight between the carelessness of my id and the reason of my ego.

I have run about eight marathons in my life, and had never hit 'the wall'. I had always finished with a sprint in around three and a quarter hours. However, I had run my last marathon nearly twenty years before, when I was younger, fitter, and four stone lighter. Standing in my fancy and expensive runners at the corner of Nassau Street as the marathon runners walked over the starting line, all I had left was my determination and my usual lunacy.

I ran the first three or four miles to the gates of the Phoenix Park at a reasonable pace. I was comfortable and measured. My back wasn't paining me and my legs were OK. My only concern was that my headache refused to go away. On the way along Pearse Street, a man of about sixty had fallen in front of me; as he tried to get up, I attempted to hurdle him and nearly broke his back and my shins. By the time I got to the first feeding station, there were already queues for the toilets for those who had chosen not to shower a wall or tree. As an Ethiopian in her togs walked back to the start, a Dubliner to my right raised a laugh when he suggested: 'Bloody elite athletes – no willpower.'

Halfway through the Park, I slowed and walked for a mile. I was beginning to feel the strain not only in my legs but also psychologically. I had aches and pains from the top of my head down to the blisters on my feet, which were itching to come out to play. It's the moment you realise you have been an idiot, and if you could only just go home, you would. My wife had made me bring the price of a bus fare in my shorts, in case the opportunity arose to jump on a bus. Getting a bus home would be a bit of a problem, though: the buses were off the roads for the duration of the marathon in the direction I was going, and if I wanted to quit I would have to walk home. I decided to make a bit of an effort and go on. Breaking into a slight jog again around Chapelizod, Inchicore and Dolphin's Barn, for a time the pain was manageable, although running on empty is about as enjoyable as eating a snack box through a straw. By the time I reached Crumlin, the race had already been won, and I was now in bits psychologically as well as physically. The idea of stealing a bike became a real possibility. Unfortunately, residents along the marathon route must have suffered this problem in the past, for bikes, along with buses and cars, were in short supply.

By the halfway mark, I had found a bit more resolution and was walking my way to a six-hour finish. At Fosters Avenue, a Canadian runner told her friend that she would never again complain about bad sex. I struggled painfully through the last six miles, not able to stop, but not really able to go on either, my poor sore legs and lower body in need of a transplant. Above the waist was fine and, entering the last bend, I let rip and sprinted across the tape. My time was clocked at 6 hours, 30 minutes and 55 seconds – a muppet's time. It was twice as slow as my previous worst time, twenty-odd years before. Most of the crowd had already dispersed, and I was grateful that no one shouted: 'Hey, fat bloke, do I know you from somewhere?' Having collected my medal – even the losers get mementos – the Conscience arrived with the car and we went home. Physically, I was bollocksed, and I knew it would take my feet a couple of months to recover from the severe blistering they had received. As I sat relaxing in a hot bath, my wife gave me a cold beer. It nearly killed me: I became all hot and bothered after a few swigs, and I had to jump out of the bath and sit by a window until I'd calmed down. It felt like post-traumatic stress and dehydration brought on by trying to rehydrate with beer. *Fuck*, I said to myself, *I won't do that again* – not really sure whether I was referring to the marathon or the beer.

November

The Wife, The Conscience and Childhood
or Can You Lose Weight in a Spa?

Almost from the moment we started dating, my wife has always been my weight conscience – governing and overseeing what I eat, don't eat, or want to eat. In some ways, she is like the classic mahout – the elephant driver – manoeuvring the big fat bloke from one meal to the next, with as little fuss as possible, always in the direction leading away from fast food. As we're at such close quarters, there's not an inch of food that goes into my mouth that she doesn't see, hear, smell or feel. Fourth, fifth, sixth senses, she's got them all – and is a right little Nancy Drew in food-police circles. There is literally nothing I eat that I can hide from her – at least not for long.

So interested is she in my welfare that she regularly turns my study upside down – during regular shakedowns – searching for the contraband of biscuits, cake, chocolate and sweets that I may have hidden behind the bookcases, files and reminder piles. Her nose is so good on these occasions that for a long time I have believed that, if the prison service ever gave her a part-time detective job clearing the jails of drugs, mobile phones, and listeners to Joe Duffy's radio programme, it would only take her a week to change Irish society. But hey, that's why a conscience is a conscience, looking out for you, even when you don't want looking out for. And, sure if the Conscience wasn't looking out for me, who would?

Most of the time, I try my best not to let on if I've had a snack box or a sly pizza, in essence pulling the wool over the Conscience's eyes. What the Conscience doesn't know won't hurt her, I tell myself. However, she being my conscience, the communication lines for the most part are honest. Too bloody honest, to be honest. In fact, what lets me down more than any other of my less attractive traits is my ability to confess. The same power refuses to allow me the luxury to hold secrets, certainly not for long. Like, what's that all about? It's obsessional in itself, almost always wanting to tell, eager to reveal my secret stash, always willing to own up. (In food terms only, you understand: I'm not a complete wimp.) The only problem is that, while I'm giving up all these confessions, I do wish – and I know that I'm very close to achieving it – that I could just give up what I spend all my days confessing to. How stupid is that? Like, why would a grown man confess to his wife that he's pigged out during the day or that he's eaten his way through a large box of chocolates? There's definitely a thesis there for some bright psychology student. I for one don't know what causes me to be so confessional. Do I want to be caught? I don't think so. It's probably got something to do with the conscience thing: admitting things is all part of the process.

Not that there hasn't been heartbreak along the way. Once, in the south of France, we had a bit of a tiff – this is confessional as well – over whether it was a good idea to turn off the motorway for chips. Starved of fast food for days, I lost it and drove into a well-known fast-food restaurant without getting her agreement and, leaving the Conscience in the car, stormed in for my dinner. Unfortunately, I made a bit of a show of myself. By some fluke of bad luck, I inadvertently pressed the remote control on my car keys and locked the poor Conscience in the car. No sooner was I in the queue to place my order than an irate Frenchwomen accosted me for caging the wife in the jalopy. You can forget Bertie having to explain what he did with the £30,000 to renovate his rented accommodation – the Conscience has never believed anything other than her opinion, which I reject, that I locked her in the car in anger so that I could selfishly feed myself on chips. However, unlike Bertie, I have always remained resolute in my unchanging story, Conscience or no Conscience.

Nearly all the time, however, the Conscience does her best to keep me on the straight and narrow, curbing my unhealthy appetite with tasty, proper food, reheating my soup (something I can't bear, as I've said previously), and encouraging me to take the healthy option. It can't be easy for a woman living with a fat bloke like me, with enough obsessional peculiarities to keep a psychiatry wing in a minor hospital in employment for the next twenty years, and who would eat chips off your sore leg if that's all there was left for dinner. And that's all before I get to my regular rant of 'I have nothing to wear' every time we get invited to a do or drinks out, when invariably I end up blaming the Conscience for everything being against me. While I sit there in my jocks, pondering whether I should go in my birthday suit or put up with the breathtakingly tight blue shirt and trousers which allow no circulation, the conversation inevitably turns to diets that have failed, and the usual confessions.

Yes, I'm sorry that I gorged myself when I had the opportunity not to. Yes, I know I'm a bloody pig, and yes, you're right when you say I should have listened to you. And yes, I know that snack box last night with the extra portion of chips was a mistake, but what's that got to do with finding a comfortable shirt and trousers to wear, now, to the theatre (or the pub). Jesus, it's a big enough conundrum to frighten the bejaysus out of King Solomon. What would Solomon have done in the circumstances – threaten to divide the snack box and extra portion of chips in half between himself and God knows who?

Not that you'd expect Solomon to answer the riddle, since many kings have come unstuck on the topic of food. In Greek mythology, Tantalus, son of Zeus and father of Niobe and Pelops, is remembered as the one who, after a disagreement with the 'authorities', was sent to Hades, where, as a punishment, he was left to stand in water up to his chin and was 'tantalised' with food and water, which moved out of his range every time he reached for them. It's a bit like the trick you play on your little brother when you're dragooned into babysitting him. For his troubles, of course, it was poor thirsty and hungry Tantalus, the patron saint of dieters, who gave his name to Victorian wine and spirit decanters, those locked cupboards of alcohol that laughed out from the shiny glass as the working servants did their rounds. Tantalus, while never the ancient world's equivalent of Ronnie Biggs or the Krays, did steal ambrosia – not rice, you understand – from the gods. He also killed his son Pelops, threw him into his biggest pot and then served him to the gods in a stew at a special feast. Cleverly, the gods – except Demeter, the hungry hoor, who absent-mindedly ate part of the boy's shoulder – recognised the liver, legs and tongue, took pity on the boy and brought him back to life. Now there's a trick that would restore your faith in Paul Daniels – not a lot, but you'll like it.

On the subject of kingly diets, historically, the great and the famous have never done well. Take, for instance, William the Bastard – or, as the English prefer to describe him, William the Conqueror. Having fought off his enemies on the way to the English crown, he then let himself go, sat around like Marlon Brando eating ice cream all day in front of his court, didn't take regular exercise, and piled on enormous amounts of weight. The French king Philip I commented – not surprisingly, considering that he wanted the 'Bastard' out of France – that William looked 'just like a pregnant woman'. (When I went to my doctor to complain that I had irritable pain in my side, I got similar advice, along the lines of: 'Paul, your body thinks you're pregnant.') Anyway, one day, washing his face in the Thames, William caught sight of himself in the river – a fat bloke who had let himself go – and nearly fell in with the fright. This wasn't the king who had mastered the English, he thought to himself, and so he immediately went to his bedroom, locked himself in, like Howard Hawkes, the aviator and film producer – another ice-cream junkie with a food obsession – refused food, and drank only alcohol, probably including the Heineken that the Danes had just arrived with from Scandinavia. However, like every poor sod who embarks on a diet, there's never the isolation of your own conviction. And so while poor William was trying desperately to trim his burgeoning body, his generals came to his bedroom and told him that the French garrison at Mantes had made a raid into Normandy, and was now acting the maggot and needed seeing to. So, William left his diet and legged it – actually he was carried by his army – to Rouen, where, in the debris of the Siege of Mantes in 1087, he received abdominal injuries from his saddle pommel when he fell off a horse. He died at the convent of St Gervais. As usual, fat people, who suffer so much indignity in life, also suffer in death. In William's case, the funeral director had last measured his body for the sarcophagus after the Battle of Hastings, twenty-one years earlier, and of course, his obese body wouldn't fit the original tomb. So instead of the usual outpouring of pain and sorrow, the chief mourners, bishops, assembled congregation and a garrison of soldiers took turns to heave the corpulent body into its final resting place. Funeral-directorship wasn't what it is today, though, and the body burst, releasing in death what the king had so desperately failed to liberate in life, dispersing the mourners from the chapel as the death fumes and other sundries announced: 'Jesus, what's that smell? Is the king dead? Jesus, long live the king.'

Incidentally, fat people haven't had the luckiest times on horses, with many having the fatal habit of falling off them. Genghis Khan fell off his horse and died – another example, if one was needed, that fat people should stay the fuck away from animals unless they're eating them. One of the only times a horse is useful is when you're getting your portrait on a horse painted, provided that the painter's in your pocket and he's prepared to paint you thin. For instance, take a look at the Bayeux Tapestry – the eleventh-century *Hello!* – the next time you're in Normandy, and see for yourself how concerned the thin Bastard was about his appearance when it was decided to commission a piece of cloth seventy metres long by half a metre wide to record the shenanigans, subterfuge and embryonic Machiavellianism that led to the Battle of Hastings in 1066. Beside the other protagonists – Edward the Confessor and Earl Harold of Wessex – William the Conqueror looks anorexic, up to and including his victory over 'perfidious Harold'. Proving that behind every fat bloke there's a conscience, or a wife. William is, in some ways, historically overshadowed by his wife, Matilda of Flanders. Despite the argument 'It's an embroidery, not a tapestry, stupid', the Bayeux Tapestry tells William's story through the eyes and ears of his wife – what you might call his conscience. It is no coincidence that the French refer to the tapestry as *La Tapisserie de la Reine Mathilde*. Does this explain why William appears thin in the famous embroidery? Not that he is the only fat-bloke reference in the cloth's history. During the Second World War, while Hitler's orders to destroy Paris in 1944 stood, Himmler, apparently, sent two emissaries to France to salvage this primary account of Britain's last conquest by a foreign army – to show Göring that even kings could be thin.

Not that William is the only king to deserve a throne in fat-bloke's heaven. His son Henry I died in 1135 of food poisoning, having eaten what history famously records as a 'a surfeit of lampreys' – eels, to you and me, which the king ate with as much frequency as I would a snack box – at Saint-Denis-en-Lyons (now Lyons-la-Forêt) in Normandy. Like his father before him, his remains were stuffed into a receptacle: in Henry's case, his corpse was unceremoniously sewn into the hide of a bull to preserve it for the journey home to England, until he was buried at Reading Abbey. One presumes that everyone was aware that the bull was a coffin and not dinner. And William and Henry were not the only ones to suffer in death. When Dr Robert Atkins, he of the carbodiets, died in 2003, newspaper obituary writers nearly fell over themselves reporting that the millionaire diet-promoter in fact weighed 260 pounds (more than 18 stone) on his death.

Getting back to the Conscience, my wife and I are a little odd, probably, by today's standards, in that we do a lot together. Car journeys, picnics, the pictures, the theatre, restaurants, holidays, exercising, gardening and cooking – we do them all together, side by side. Sometimes it gets a little claustrophobic, particularly when I'm driving, as it feels like we're driving by committee. Hands up who wants to turn left? One hand – mine. Hands up who wants to turn right? One hand – the Conscience. We turn right. OK, so who said democracy was going to be easy? Anyway, we had planned to go to a spa to see if this could help me lose weight. Yeah, I know, it sounds ridiculous, but hey, I'm desperate, and I'll try anything at least once. So we booked the spa and put the plans in motion. Unfortunately, the Conscience at the last minute couldn't make it, due to unforeseen work commitments, and so I went down for the day by myself.

There's something peculiarly Irish about sitting in an outdoor hot tub in Wicklow in the middle of autumn in lashings of rain, the dark-grey clouds trumpeting the prologue to winter. But there I was at the Brooklodge and Wells Spa Centre at Macreddin village in County Wicklow, naked except for my swimming togs and goggles, and crouched on my hunkers in a barrel-shaped wooden bowl – which could easily have housed The Old Woman Who Lived in a Shoe and at least four of her children if she had a mind to seek other accommodation – the warm comfort of heated water gently tidal-waving that spiky part around my neck where I often forget, or hate, to shave. As the rain got heavier, I submerged myself, the rain tip-toeing 'Top Hat' on the part of my head which hovered an inch or two above sea level. Down below, my goggles tight to my eyes, I closed my winkers and imagined the tranquillity of nothingness. Back up above, I realised that tight haircuts – I'd had my hair cut the day before –are only any good on someone with a long neck. Otherwise, a person like me looks like one of the Bash Street Kids, particularly the one with the spots, or a toadstool that's been squashed into someone else's bum.

Earlier that morning, I had arrived at the prearranged time of 9.30 AM, having made my way down in the driving rain. After being met at reception, I was given the tour – pool, relaxation rooms, steam room, changing rooms – handed a white bathrobe and slippers, and told to relax and take my time, get to know the place, change into my whites and take in a swim if I wanted to. At 10.30 AM I should make my way to the waiting room, where a masseur would summon me for my massage. So, changed, robed, relaxed and ensconced in one of those elongated deckchairs that resemble the outline of a half-cut swastika, I arrived early for my appointment. Not to worry, I said to myself, take it all in, get your thoughts on an even keel, sleep a little, think of the poor wife slaving over her workstation, and relax, relax, relax. Unfortunately, the waiting room – an open and busy space – was a little chilly. Not that I, or anybody else, was complaining. Most were gripping their whites a little closer, accepting that the residue from a long, warm summer had probably made the heat switch on the heating redundant, notwithstanding that the morning in question was a day on which the dove wouldn't have left the Ark.

The waiting room itself was Masonic in design, and the circular ceiling, marble floor and diffuse medieval-style lighting gave it the resonance of a Knights Templar chapel that had recently been decorated. Except for the modernity of blue-lit bubbles on the wall behind me, which followed other bubbles like champagne suds on manoeuvres (and were enough to make me thirsty) and the woman opposite me, who had obviously brought a year's supply of perfume with her, I expected *The Da Vinci Code*'s Robert Langdon to come running in, screaming that there had been a murder. The Brooklodge is too subtle for that, though; the only disturbance for the other guests was my presence: I was the sole man, and thus the only fat bloke, among fourteen others in a parlour which, to my mind, was more commonly associated with the fairer sex. Later, I'm told that 20 percent of all clients to the lodge are men – a coterie of businessmen, builders and ordinary bods – swapping other diversions for the pampering.

At 10.30, the masseur, Ludo, introduces himself and leads me to the massage room. I follow, energised from three-quarters of an hour of people-watching. Ludo puts me on my stomach, my face lying over the bed in a sling-like head-support, and asks me if I'm amenable to his 'particularly hard type of massage – it's good, no?' I agree, not wanting to appear weak, letting him know that I have a bad back and a touch of sciatica that won't go away; the sort of excuses, although valid, that have enough credit to give me an out if my pain threshold is reached.

We begin, and immediately it's a mixture of the Dam Busters (specifically Sir Barnes Wallace's bouncing bomb), Bruce Lee chopping carrots, and the ramming-speed test-drive from *Ben Hur*. I'm clenching my teeth as the masseur goes up and down my spine from my neck to my lower buttocks on the first part of the massage. I huff and aaggh and moan and curse; the masseur is oblivious to all of this, and for a solid half an hour introduces my spinal cord to boot-camp. It's not exactly lingeringly painful in an Amnesty International sort of way, but I'm desperately grateful

I'm not on rendition, and let's get this straight, while I don't actually cry, I count the minutes to the end. When he's finished, Ludo tells me that my back might be sore tomorrow or the next day and that, really, a man of my proportions should go for a massage once a week. If only, Ludo, if only – I'd probably have more luck throwing a pair of sixes.

The second part of the treatment is a head massage. For this, I sit up at the side of the bed as Ludo runs his fingers, knuckles and fist nearly through my neck and head. It's very invasive, and particularly uncomfortable around my neck, where recently I've had a bit of a crick. It's painful, as my log-jammed Red Cow roundabout of a neck starts to unwind, presumably freeing the various nerves to go their separate ways. By the time it's all over, I've been nearly an hour in the masseur's company, and I feel a lot less tight around my back and neck, and have probably lost about three pounds. I want to go and weigh myself, but can't find a scales. I decide to go for a swim instead.

The pool is mine except for the odd hotel guest who has dropped in for a quick swim, a go in the jacuzzi or the sauna, or just to read a novel at the water's edge in the seating provided. I swim a few lengths before braving the pelting rain and the great outdoors of the hot tub. *Ah*, I say to myself, *this is the life*, my goggles high on my head. From a couple of thousand feet – if, God forbid, someone had the mind to invade us from the air – a fighter pilot would have thought it was Biggles taking a dip.

Another swim later, it was lunchtime – a little more substantial than a big salad, but not enough to convince me not to stop off for a snack box on the way home in future. By the time I had finished my dessert, it was only two o'clock, and I had another two hours to kill before my facial appointment. So, to chill out a little further, I went into the relaxation room, where the blinds keep out the natural light and candlelight provides the therapeutic equivalent of night-vision. I counted five women in the room. Once more on my back, this time with earphones, I closed my eyes and listened to a poor man's version of *Tubular Bells*. Sleep came slowly, but soon I was deep in some murder mystery, until I thought I could hear myself snoring, and, embarrassed, dragged myself up one of those imaginary ladders to consciousness. Awake, I was now alone in the room, probably having cleared it with the snoring.

Like most men, a facial is uncharted waters for me. I wasn't sure what I was getting, and not really sure where the benefits would be felt. The last time I let anyone near my face to clean it was back in the days when my mother would embarrassingly spit into her hankie and try to add a shine to my dirty face when I was in primary school. So there I was, lying on my back, getting my first aromaplastie facial, the low background music putting me to sleep again, my 'therapist' standing behind me, making up the potions for the clean-up. The treatment began. A double milk cleanse, followed by a deep cleanse and an exfoliation. And a pressure point and drainage massage with rose oil, followed by an wheat-germ mask. My therapist is talking me through what's happening. New words fly past like F-16s – 'emulsion creams', 'hydra floras', 'essentials oils' and 'peels'. I'm not sure if they're brand names, designer labels or shortcuts in the trade. I do recognise the odd phrase, like 'cleansing water', 'toner', 'moisturiser' and 'mask', but don't ask me to explain what they do or don't do. By this time, my nostrils are performing somersaults adjusting to the many fragrances and oils that are sweeping over my face, from scented oranges to the aroma of walking in an autumn forest. My therapist covers my face in light bandaging, like you'd imagine someone trying to hide the Invisible Man. Underneath, with patches protecting my eyes, and my face staring up at a white sky, my therapist asks in a whisper (conscious that I might not be) would I like a hand, arm or foot massage. I ask for a recommendation. She suggests the foot massage. I suddenly realise that my toenails look like battle-hardened velociraptors, are in sorry need of a crew-cut and might not be as presentable as I'd like for their massaging debut. Before I've time to change my mind, though, she's hard at work playing with my feet, tickling all the right nerves. It's happy days, and great to be alive. The foot massage out of the way, she peels the mask from my face, toning and massaging as she goes, adding a little aftershave balm for good measure. By 5.30 PM I'm up, dressed and back in the car for the steady drive home. Am I any better off for the experience? Probably. Would I do it again? Probably not. Have I lost any weight? Possibly around my face, neck and shoulders. Would I need a weighing scales to measure it? Probably not.

DECEMBER

CHRISTMAS PARTIES, THE PERSONAL TRAINER AND THE WHIFF OF SUCCESS

December is normally a reasonably easy four- or five-odd weeks for a fat bloke. It's usually a lot colder, and with the hours of daylight countable on the fingers of one hand, it's one of the best months for hiding fat under the cloak of heavy clothing and darkness. It's also a month where it is much more sociably acceptable to let yourself go, knowing that a new beginning is only around the corner in the New Year. Eating, overeating and piling on the weight suddenly become a mission statement, and a national obsession. Fat-blokeism goes global. It's also traditionally the month the food police go into hibernation, far too busy putting up the decorations or out buying presents to worry if your trousers are too tight or whether you're going to go with the blue shirt this Christmas, for the fifth, or is it the sixth, year in a row. That is, of course, assuming that your treads still have a shelf life and that you haven't allowed your body mass to explode. Otherwise, you're courting the disaster of shopping for seasonal clobber at the wrong time of the year.

Not surprisingly, food-wise, Christmas has always been a disaster for me, and the lead-up to it poses a perennial conundrum: why the fuck can't I arrive at the end of that third week of December, after a year of pain trying to lose a few inches, having made some effort to cut down on the usual junk and other atrocities that sabotage any semblance of dietary constraint or efforts at weight loss? The problem, however, is that the festive season is on top of me before I have time to worry about it, and I'm already lost trying to avoid the Christmas-party season by the time the invitations arrive. The ability to avoid such parties is probably the Third Secret of Fatima. Like, what are you going to say when the invitations arrive? 'Oh, I'm really, really sorry, but do you remember me telling you for the last ten years that I have a fucking weight problem that puts me on the Christmas-party danger list? Like, do you want trouble? Well, what the hell are you playing at sending me another invitation?' It's really, really difficult, and no amount of hindsight prepares you for it. You just hope the invitations don't arrive, but of course they do. They are like summonses to a slow death, and it's reason enough to lose weight. In the end, you just go, ritualistically, to see which plonker, this year, will make a fool of himself, and whether the usual rules of engagement are being enforced, but it's by no means an ultra-happy journey.

For the last two thousand years, the ethics and rules governing Christmas parties have shared the same DNA, and often the same bed, from Constantinople to Temple Bar. Pure and simple: don't bring to the mayhem your wife, husband, girlfriend, boyfriend, dog or photocopier. Don't expect to get home before dawn, don't expect to get a taxi, and don't expect any sympathy for your ensuing hangover. In fact, don't expect anything, just let it happen, and remember that Christmas parties are for losers. Expect to lose your inhibitions, dignity, respect, money, voice, shirt, tie, knickers, virginity, marriage, and possibly job. And if you're with Bruce Willis, expect to be separated from your shoes, vest, blood, escalators, mercenaries, long-haired brother, English-German dictionary, windows, patrol car and possibly accommodation. The Romans knew it, the Carthaginians knew it, and now you know it.

So why attend these annual mortification-fests of debauchery, unruliness and abandonment? Well, maybe you just enjoy the embarrassment, excessive drinking, group-hugs, inter-departmental bitching, bad food and cheap wine, and the opportunity to behave as though you're attending the Wesley disco for the first time. Or maybe you're the fat bloke in the corner, helping himself to extra spuds, gravy, and turkey and ham. Or maybe, because you're on such a tight leash at home or even at work – deprived of all the creature comforts your subconscious craves, including food – any opportunity to subvert authority, the establishment, the house rules or your ordinary morals releases your id and provides it with enough testosterone and wherewithal to charm the entire secretarial pool into re-enacting the Battle of the Boyne in the boss's secret mudbath on the top floor.

Or maybe you're a boring fat bloke and it's because it's the only opportunity in the calendar you get to chin-wag with Britney in Accounts or Malcolm in IT, or to press the flesh of the company's lesser-known ambassadors. Or maybe it's because you just love listening to boring Brian tell his long, long, long list of 1970s Christmas jokes just one more time. Or maybe you just want to hear if Michael is now Mary in Junior Admin or whether Danielle is Daniel in Credit Risk. Or maybe you're planning a coup and/or a leadership challenge and you just want to network with the troops to gauge the potential opposition. Or maybe you figure it's a good time to tell your work colleagues that times are hard, that you're planning to leave the wife for a chipper in Enniscorthy, that you're short of readies, and would they mind passing around the Leeds United half-centenary plate once more for old times' sake.

Whatever you're thinking, your boss is never far from your thoughts. Unlike any other night out with the boss – from stag weekends to hen nights – where the boss is just another drunk on the prowl, another seat in the dentist's chair, the end-of-year bash is different. At the Christmas party, they're undoubtedly the Generalissimo, the First Lady, Il Duce, the Iron Lady, Top Cat, the all-powerful Zeus, the doppelgänger Jupiter, or even Napoleon. They are there to share their gravitas, virtue, time, generosity, good cheer, airspace, will-to-power, wisdom, body odours and poor-Oxfam dress sense.

They are the ones you have to be wary of, the ones you don't want to see you knocking the angel off the Christmas tree with a half-eaten margarined baguette, or with his face stuck in a bowl of cream. Within their grasp, they hold your fledgling career, promotional prospects, company car, an understanding of your expense sheets, and any follow-through on the promise of a New Year pay rise. And past performance is no guarantee of future rewards. Everything hangs on your performance at *this* Christmas party: how you hold your knife and fork, and how you deal with the cocktails, the wine, the Irish coffees, the cheese board, the insanely drunk and available dictation temp, and most importantly of all, your mouth.

The sitting arrangements are paramount. While the snivellers, office pets and sycophants mug the space around the boss, jockeying for their attention while not necessarily wanting to sit on their lap, you should at least be within eye contact, across the table and slightly upstream if possible. You want to be close enough to be noticed but not too close to be a nuisance. Or worse still, to be heard. You want to be a trusted lieutenant of the Grand Armée – Ney, Davout, Dano, Mutley or Cowen – and a person of undoubted elegance and depth. And considered by many in the know to have the ear of the Chosen One, closer to the Teflon than the Teflon itself. The sort of disciple that could be trusted not to take home or sell off the loaves and the fishes: the voice of good sense when the old badgers start fighting over the young skirts or when Sales kick up a fuss with Distribution, or when the swingers in your own department start networking and talking shop with New Acquisitions.

You, an all-round company diehard, are one of the crew, the junta's eyes and ears if they want them, a solid pints drinker and a favourite of the masses. You are only out for a good time, a few drinks, the joy of socialising, and a bit of craic, conscious that one of the main reasons for exchanging presents at Christmas is saying sorry for your performance at the Christmas do. If you use your mouth for a living, hang out with trainspotters or work with people who name hurricanes, my thoughts are that your favourite conversation is silence, and the annual jamboree to the end-of-season nosh-up is causing you sleepless nights. Or, embedded with super-bores, vocabulary terrorists, and soap-anoraks, you live in hope that the spook in the entertainment department gets a personality transplant and organises the Christmas party in a monastery, Zen retreat or cave in Afghanistan, where a thin bloke in a white overshirt is preparing Osama's GI Diet – and no, it's not duck.

My record at the company Christmas party, however, is pretty abysmal. I was once the last person to be served in a well-known Dublin hotel, only to be told that they had run out of turkey and ham, and would I mind more spuds. 'Are you out of your fucking mind?' I'd asked. 'It's the Christmas do, for Christ's sake, how the fuck could you run out of turkey and ham.' 'Sorry, sir, we budgeted for 1,010 people and you're number 1,011 – would you prefer roast potatoes?'

And of course, there was the occasion when I was invited to the annual gathering on the same day the company sacked me. Not to my face, you understand. No, the cowards – who for legal reasons shall remain nameless – sent me a cheesy letter written with all the usual highfalutin' borrowed aphorisms that complicate a simple situation. So badly ghost-written was it that Marley's ghost and Ebenezer Scrooge would have run out of Christmases before I knew what the letter was saying, and why. It took ten or twelve readings, and a further five consultations, to establish that yes, I was being shafted. Yes, shafted in Christmas week. So there I was, Monday morning, Bob 'without-a-job' Cratchit, reading a notice terminating the contract I didn't have, arriving in work expecting some sort of recognition from management that this was my last week in the office, only to discover that I'd been invited to the Christmas party.

Needless to say, I went, pretended to be outrageously drunk; slagged everybody off from a height; ordered obscenely the dearest drinks on the menu; told the general manager that I for one wasn't going to ignore the fact that his hair wasn't real; that yes, it was me who'd over-ordered on the staples and treasury tags; that Joannie on the switch was going to report him for harassment; and that his wife was having an affair with Fred, the fork-lift driver. As I was manhandled from the premises by four security guards, he shouted after me: 'I'm going to sack you first thing tomorrow morning.' 'Sack me twice. Who ever heard of that?' I laughed back. 'And furthermore, about my reference – put it in the post, will yeh?' You can't beat a bit of impunity at the Christmas party, can you?

At another Christmas party in Powers Hotel in Kildare Street about twenty years ago, after we ran out of buns to throw, the mood dropped so low it could have gone out with the Liffey tide, a street or two down. Bored, I called my friends at home and told them I was leaving soon and would see them for some serious partying. However, an hour or two later, with more drink on board, I rang them again to say that things had cheered up immensely. I told them – and I can't for the life of me say why – that during the meal I had requested duck. When informed that duck was not on the menu, I volunteered to go out and fetch one. I then told my friends that, while in the course of strangling a duck in the dark in St Stephen's Green, I was arrested by the Guards, charged with the unlawful attempted murder of a species known or unknown, and brought to Store Street Garda Station. I concluded that everything was being sorted out and that I'd be home soon. This, of course, was all a massive lie.

Back home, my friends took matters into their own hands and called into my mother and told her what had happened, and that she wasn't to worry. When she pointed out that this was possibly a wind-up, they embellished the story with talk of rumours of a lengthy sentence and prison. As you can imagine, my poor mother was out of her wits with worry. They then sped off, got their father out of bed – they were obviously too drunk to drive, even in those drink-driving days – and headed for Store Street. In the station, the duty sergeant told them that if I had been arrested in St Stephen's Green, I had more than likely been taken to Pearse Street Garda Station. At Pearse Street, after the duty sergeant had been convinced that it wasn't a wind-up, he took them on a tour of the cells, pointing out that none of those incarcerated came in wet – wet in the sense that they might have been swimming in St Stephen's Green – or were in possession of a duck, whether dead or alive. He also pointed out that most of his prisoners were so drunk that they weren't able to give their names. Realising that I wasn't among the casualties, they returned to Store Street, where, after a tour of the cells, they proceeded on to Kevin Street,

Donnybrook, Fitzgibbon Street, the Bridewell and Mountjoy, before going on to the hospitals. At 5 AM they gave up, returning home demoralised and angry, reporting to my besieged mother the run of events, and that I was now officially AWOL.

By the time I arrived home, it was close to 6 AM. My mother met me at the door, grasping for wetness in my clothes and wondering 'What time did you get out?' 'Get out,' says I. 'From where?' 'From the police station,' says she. 'You were locked up for strangling a duck in St Stephen's Green.' At that stage, events came back to haunt me, as my mother recalled how the situation had unfolded in my absence and how I had savagely hoodwinked my friends. To this day, my friends still believe that I did strangle a duck in St Stephen's Green, that I was arrested, and that by some incredible stroke of genius I was able to pull strings to effect my release. I've always maintained that they should have seen it coming, and that someone should have shouted 'Duck!'

That all gets away from the fact that eleven months into my major plan to lose weight, and all set for the Christmas-party season, all my best plans have ended in failure. Not complete failure, mind: I am down a stone in weight. Nevertheless, if you consider that, before this year, I have put on a stone a year for the last five years, I could at least prosper in the long run, if I could lose a stone a year for the next four years as well. However, despite all my efforts – I can't really call them my *best* efforts – I am still a slave to fast food, and all the other food-related goodies. So, as one last effort to finish the year on a high, I have employed a personal trainer to help me gradually back into my running, the disaster of the marathon an aberration in the past. Extreme? Yes. Ultimately, I'm paying someone to be my friend, to go running with me. It's sad-bastard territory, and I'm not particularly happy about it.

The first time I meet the personal trainer, Matthew, I read that a recent piece of research from the *New England Journal of Medicine* suggests that obesity is contagious. Matthew is as thin as a rake: gaunt, you might say, even unhealthy and undernourished. I sense that putting the research to the test will prove conclusively that whoever is financing the *New England Journal of Medicine*'s research had more money than sense. The first night, Matthew calls to my house, and I sign all sorts of waivers, exonerating the trainer of any guilt in the event of my death or serious injury. It's not the confidence-boost I was expecting, but hey, he's only protecting his own interests, and sure I'm a grown man anyway. I'm weighed, and my body-fat percentage, body-fat mass, fat-free mass, body-mass index and the amount of water in my system is calculated. The scales give all the readings, and I can't say I'm impressed by them – or care to understand them. We warm up in the kitchen. Matthew has brought along his own ghetto-blaster, and we warm up loudly, to a dance beat. The space is tight, irritable and uncomfortable, with not enough room to swing as much as one leg or arm at any one time. Twenty minutes later, we're out running – not very far, but enough to have me knackered by the time we're coming back, the pain in my back grating into my spine. But hey, twenty minutes on day one is progress: slow progress, maybe, but definitely progress.

Back in the house for the warm-down, we agree that the house is not the shape or the size for this, and we arrange to run the programme from a designated area in the Phoenix Park which is about twenty minutes from home in the car. And so, the following week, I arrive in the park ready for action. Matthew is already there, his windows rolled down, his music system blaring out disco, dance and funk, and we have an audience in tow – three women with four children – who are talking to each other in the cold air. We warm up to the beat, like rejects from *Fame*, me the fat, stupid, out-of-shape bloke with the spare tyre, and Matthew the ultra-thin training junkie who's very excited. The warm-up is embarrassing, but Matthew tells me it's really important. We dance in, we dance out. Pull the arms in, push the arms out. Jog a little this way, jog a little that way. Arms in the sky, arms by the sides. Walk in, walk out. Swing the left leg out, swing the right leg out. Crouch forward, crouch back. And all the time the music pumps up Matthew like he's going to do a Spiderman through the trees, while I on the other hand am clearly the Penguin, desperate to avoid any semblance of daylight and, more importantly, to curb my burgeoning embarrassment.

Taking a water break, I rush to the car to get my prescription sunglasses, eager to hide from prying eyes the identity of the overweight barrel who's replicating St Vitus' Dance to a Britney dance-track. This just isn't me. Yes, I was once able to shake a leg. Yes, I once thought I was Tony Manero. But for fuck's sake, I'm at least five stone over my dancing weight and look like a sack of potatoes jumping up and down. OK, so I'm supposed to be focused on a bit of training, and it *is* only warming up, but hey, we're two blokes out in the middle of the Phoenix Park in the middle of a Saturday afternoon in broad daylight, like two rejects from the YMCA, and even if no one recognises me, with good-looking women walking up and down all around me, I want to have at least some semblance of pride in who I am – or who I want to be. Dancing to music that's twenty-odd years out of my time zone with Matthew, the happiest bloke on the planet, makes me wonder if the Conscience, who recently suggested I should go and see a food shrink, is right, because she thinks that my weight problem runs much deeper than a mere love of food. It's nano-nano nano-nano territory, and not something I'm particularly comfortable with. I can only imagine going to the food shrink and telling him: 'The wife thinks my relationship with food needs a head doctor, and that I should go and talk to someone.' What's he going to say to me? 'Careful, son, getting up on that couch. I'm only insured for sixteen and a quarter stone.' Like, what could a psychologist or a psychiatrist tell me that I don't already know about my eating habits? Stop eating, hippo?

I realise very quickly that the dance-beat is never going to do it for me. It's far too lollipoppy, and doesn't come with any guitar riffs or lyrics. Christ, it's not even personal. For a warm-up, it's got more in common with Legs & Co. or a Jane Fonda workout. If anything, it's going to drive me to boiling point, never mind warming me up. And as for my embarrassment threshold over the coming months, it's going to drive my reading off the Richter scale. And yet Matty, sorry *Matthew* – he keeps telling me 'Don't call me Matty' – is terribly enthusiastic, and I don't want to burst his bubble over a few songs. So I put up with it, at least in the short term.

I'm relieved when it's time to start the actual running. We head off down the main road of the park, Chesterfield Avenue – on the cycling track (Matthew says 'It's a better surface, and sure, the cyclists won't mind') – past the Visitor Centre, the Phoenix Monument, the Áras, the Polo Grounds, the Zoo and the Wellington Monument to the Parkgate Street gate, and then back up again uphill, to where we started. It takes me an hour to go barely three kilometres, with Matthew running along beside me looking bored. *I don't pay you to be bored, Matthew, so you can change that face for a start,* I say to myself. By the end of the run, I can feel some power coming into my legs, and just completing an hour of running, without stopping, gives me a bit of a boost.

However, the bit of success hasn't been without turmoil – most of it for Matty, sorry *Matthew,* who over the course of our regular runs down the length of the Phoenix Park has to listen to my every complaint and whinge. Chief among these grievances are the pains in my Achilles heels, back, bum and calves. My Achilles seem to be taking the brunt of the aggro as I try to run moderately fast for an hour. With nearly all the action taking place in my stomach, where most of my weight is lodged – weight-wise I'm really fat around the midriff, less so on top, and definitely not in my legs – my weight seems to shift from side to side before driving a sledgehammer down though the central spine section of my spine, the pounding finally (although we're talking microseconds here) landing on the lowest part of my body, and the pressure points around my ankles, notably my Achilles. The pain is manageable save for the odd occasion when I kick myself. How do you kick yourself when running? Christ, if I knew that I'd be the dog's bollocks. However, I'm sure that Newton's thirty-fourth law of motion mentions that, when running in a straight line over a fixed distance, with a personal trainer in tow – not literally, you understand – you couldn't lay odds that some stupid fat bloke is capable of kicking his left ankle or thereabouts with his right foot. Painful? You bet it is. It makes a mockery of the old Brendan Behan joke when himself and Patrick Kavanagh are supposedly chased down Grafton Street by the Guards. Behan, with youth on his side, was able to escape over the railings of Trinity College.

Looking back, Behan could see Kavanagh on the wrong side of the railings squaring up to the Guards, his fists up like a boxer's. Says Behan: 'Fuck the Marquess of Queensberry, kick him in the bollix.' If I was in a similar position today, I would have told Kavanagh: 'Kick him in the Achilles if you really want to hurt him.'

Aside from the Achilles, the pain in my back didn't last all that long, once I started to run with a bit more frequency. In fact, over a month, the pain in my back, the one caused by my sciatica, just packed up bags and went home, never to be seen again. However, the one I think comes from the area of the liver – caused, according to any amount of expensive physicians I care to talk to, by the final stages of late-term pregnancy – has remained like one of those nosy retired types who seems to have swapped suburbia for tribunal-living, spending more time in the company of witnesses than any lawyer.

My diverticular disease, or hole trouble, has probably been my most uncomfortable experience. While I probably don't drink as much water as the Conscience – a camel among connoisseurs – I have in recent weeks started to drink gallons of water each day, to correct a problem that was noticeable in my stool, where hard acorns of discontent have replaced my regular loo-flushes of diarrhoea. Obviously, the running is drying up my water resources – stiffening up my resolve, so to speak. Which all seems pretty normal, until the hole trouble kicks in every so often when I'm trying to run. It's as if a great wedge of blockage is fortifying the Khyber Pass at my back door. I have the sensation that a discharge would be enough to wallpaper the whole of the H-Blocks if they ever had a mind to open them again. Day in, day out, the barricade is always there – there in the sense that the nerve endings sending messages to my brain are telling me 'Jesus, it's tight down there' – while a cursory inspection (a difficult operation in itself, considering my weight) shows up nothing.

Given the nature of my diverticular disease and the medical explanation that I've pockets, alleyways and culs-de-sac off my colon, I've taken to asking Matthew to carry a little plastic bag with a facecloth, now officially my emergency bum-wiper, and a few sheets of bog-roll. You can never be too careful in these situations. Chances are that one of these days I'm going to have a major evacuation, and God help me if I'm not prepared. Like, how many toilets do I pass when I'm out running in the Park? None. The biggest enclosed city park in Europe, and there are about ten toilets on around 1,700 acres, and most of *them* are in Áras an Uachtaráin. It's not as if you could run up to the door, in the middle of a jog, and ask: 'Sorry for barging in on you like this, Madam President, and apologies to the president of Kyrgyzstan, but I noticed the light on in the window and wondered could I use your toilet?' So Matthew, along with his other chore of hauling my water during my run, now carries the CSI bag. Looking like one of those tall natives who used to carry the provisions for the famous explorer travelling through the jungle looking for Tarzan or somesuch, Matthew isn't particularly happy about having to carry supplies. I assure myself that if I have to warm up like some barrel-dolly at the Folies Bergère, he can sure handle the hardship of carrying the CSI bag.

And another thing, he's beginning to really annoy me in other ways too. OK, so he's super-fit and I'm the dunce in running-class, and probably not going as fast as he would like. But occasionally, if I start to run a little too slowly, he stops running and walks beside me. *The bastard,* I say to myself, *he's really showing me up.* It's obvious that we're training together, and anyone going by us is noticing that I'm the poor relation, and obviously not able to keep up with Mr Bloody Perfect. Sometimes he even lets out a bit of patronising encouragement for an audience, like 'Well done, you're making fantastic progress. Just keep it up', so loud that Mary McAleese could hear it if she was putting out her washing. When I get really slow, particularly if we're approaching a group of people running or cycling towards us – remember, I'm a man with two bad feet from a marathon disaster, a colon problem that effectively means I'm trying to run with a poker up my arse, heels that are about to explode from the pressure, and two sore calves that I haven't had time to tell you about – he runs away from me with a burst of speed that Eamonn Coghlan could have used in the 1976 and 1980 Olympics. He's just like something you'd expect from the natives in the *Tarzan* pictures, who always seemed to run off halfway through the picture, probably with the CSI bags. It's demoralising stuff, and I just want to go home.

I don't, however, certainly not in the sense that I give up, preferring to persevere, even going to the trouble of training on my days off, driving up to the Phoenix Park for some extra running. Strangely enough, training on my own, running along the cycle track that goes the length of the Phoenix Park from the Castleknock gate to Parkgate Street, isn't without its problems – the main one being the cyclists who think they own the bloody lane. There I am minding my own business running along at a leisurely pace on a track on which you could easily fit four athletes jogging abreast, when from afar I see cyclists coming towards me. Now, not wanting to hog all the track, and conscious that I'm in their *Lebensraum*, I've made sure that I'm over to one side, almost on the grass. One particular cyclist stares me out of it from a distance. He can see me and I can see him. Even from a hundred yards away, I can see the whites of his grinding teeth, as he cycles towards me on my side of the path. It's pure hatred on a bike. At fifty yards, he's making no effort to move, sticking to his guns. I'm tempted to move across to the other side of the path, but not having enough leverage at my weight to look nonchalantly over my shoulder to see if it's safe to move lanes without getting run down by a bike coming from behind me, I stay where I am. At twenty-five yards, the cyclist is still looking at me but is making no effort to alter his direction. He's playing chicken with a stubborn seventeen-stone mass of body organs going nowhere fast. If he doesn't move to his right within the next eight seconds, he's going to hit me. I've already decided in my mind that I'm staying put, and if I have to take a hit, well, so be it. Within seconds of the biggest incident in cycle–runner road rage since the coyote tried to catch the roadrunner on a bicycle, the cyclist changes direction, screaming in my face: 'You dozy fat bastard, are you thick, do you not know this is a cycling lane?' Within another few seconds, to the muffled sound of 'You fat thick bastard', he's gone. *Beep, beep, to you too, you bastard*, I say to myself.

*

204

As the weeks went by, probably the most painful ache I had was pain in both my calf muscles. From time to time, the pain would force me to stop running, a situation that left Matthew, running up the road ahead of me, embarrassed and bewildered. Matthew isn't one for empathy, certainly not in my case, and I can sense in his mood a belief that I'm just another fat bloke adding to his problems. He does try to help me overcome my calf difficulties, suggesting that I do various exercises, like standing on the bottom step of the stairs, slowly pressing up and down, cajoling my calves to ease up on the pain. It's time-consuming and repetitive, and something from which I don't see quick results. But hey, I persevere: it's my new mission statement. And over the following three weeks I build up a bit of stamina, and the weight begins to fall off slowly, and I'm down another stone to sixteen and a half stone, the first time I've been at that weight in three years; for my money, this is a remarkable achievement. It's beginning to sound like a little success story, and I still have the whole of next year to look forward to.

Close to Christmas, and going into the New Year, I have lost two stone over the course of the last twelve months. It's not a huge amount, but not something to turn your nose up at either. To be fair to my headspace, department policy is now firmly in favour of weight loss, proper diet and proportionality – at least most of the time. I seem to be eating a lot healthier and am certainly happier in myself, although I could never say I've cured myself of my love of bad food. Up in the attic where my mind hangs out, my identity is no longer the cheerleader for fast food, even if it struggles to keep the cravings in check. Midnight feasts and reliance on chocolate, shortbread and even almond icing are worms which I've left safely in the past. I've decided to train properly with my personal trainer – if we don't kill each other first – for next year's marathon, and to put together a proper exercise programme that will continue to be my main saving grace. At the end of a long year on weight-patrol, it might not be everyone's idea of a diet, but it's one man's Irishman's Diet – at least until the next time.